REVIEWERS &

"Very informative and motivating. From introducing the science of what goes into making health decisions to practical applications of this science, everyone can benefit from incorporating these principles into one's life. I definitely recommend this for everyone's "must read" list."

—John Pauls, M.D., Ph.D.

"Through this unassuming guide to wellness, Dr. Scher provides professional guidance that effectively promotes change in habits and routine to live a healthier life. His book is a tremendous opportunity to redefine your life. Learn to embrace your best self and your life's journey. Let this book be your guide!"

—Eryn Ann Bannister, Doctor of Physical Therapy

"Dr Scher's trend-bucking book provides an honest, straightforward and comprehensive framework for health. I think the book is really all anyone needs to get healthy, Honestly, there weren't too many surprises in this book, at least for me. You also may know a lot of what is in this book. But what you know is worthless until you put it into action, and that's where this book excels. Dr. Scher gives you discrete chunks of eminently doable tasks each week, which prevents you from becoming overwhelmed and giving up."

—Editor/Physician, HormonesDemystified.com

"Your Best Health Ever! cuts through the confusing medical language and healthcare jargon and allows readers to get to the root of what is ailing them in an easy-to-understand way. Dr. Scher's medical background as a doctor and educator coupled with his personal practice of a healthy and active lifestyle will help readers gain their "Best Health Ever." I highly recommend this book to anyone looking for a new and clear path to better health."

—Cynthia Muchnick, educator

Ordering Information

Special discounts are available on quantity purchases by corporations, associations, and others. For details, contact the publisher at the address above.

Printed in the United States of America

First Printing 2017

ISBN 978-0-692-85281-1

www.DrBretScher.com

DISCLAIMER

Information in this book is provided for informational purposes only and is not intended as a substitute for the advice provided by your physician or other healthcare professional. You should not use this book alone to diagnose or treat a health problem, or as advice to start or stop any medication or other treatment.

Opinions expressed in this book are mine alone and are not meant to represent those of any group or organization with which I am affiliated.

DEDICATION

This book is dedicated to all my mentors and teachers—those who helped instill in me the joy of learning, and the power to realize I can make a difference in people's lives by helping them learn to be better. Dr. Stan Amundson, the late Dr. Ted Heffernan, Dr. Ada Wolfson and my other colleagues at Scripps Mercy residency program. Dr. Mimi Guarneri, Dr. Dave Rubenson and other mentors and teachers in the Scripps Clinic cardiology fellowship program.

And, of course, to my family. My wife and two sons, who teach me what is truly important in life, and who inspire me to be better every day. And my parents, whose unconditional love and support helped make me who I am today.

Thank you all!

CONTENTS

ABOUT BRET SCHER, M.D.

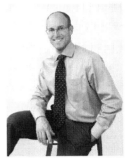

I admit it: I am a card-carrying preventive cardiologist. But if you're expecting me to recommend a fistful of prescriptions or surgery to help you reach your best health ever, you're in for a pleasant surprise.

(Unless, of course, you enjoy funding the healthcare industry.)

Like many of you, when I was growing up I never had to worry about my health, or my weight, or fitness, or what I ate. My dad always worked out, and as a kid, I'd tag along to the gym with him. As time passed, I moved on from gym workouts to cycling, swimming, running, and by my twenties, competing in Ironman triathlons before they were even popular.

Then, real life happened. I graduated from Stanford University and entered Ohio State University's medical school, followed by my internal medicine residency and a fellowship in cardiology at Scripps Clinic under Dr. Mimi Guarneri's direction.

Those gym visits, long runs and bike rides became a struggle to maintain. Finding time to eat well, stay active, get enough sleep, and handle the stress of a high-stakes job became a constant presence in my life.

At the same time, working with Dr. Guarneri accelerated the transformation of my thinking about medicine. I began to see new ways to combine cardiology and preventive medicine into the emerging specialty of integrative medicine. This approach treats the patient as a whole person, not just a collection of risk factors.

When I established my own cardiology practice as part of a large, well-known health system in San Diego a few years later, I saw the difficulties we all face in leading healthy lives and the consequences that result. It was clear to me that our healthcare system is full of people suffering from completely preventable diseases.

Suddenly, I had a clear mission: to empower all my patients to help themselves, by making the best-informed choices possible about everything from food to activity to sleep to stress management, every single day. After all, the best way to "treat" someone is to prevent the need for treatment in the first place.

I've since studied extensively in the areas of functional medicine, personal fitness training, and nutrition, adding those certifications to my credentials as a physician. That broadened my perspective, inspiring the development of the six building blocks that form the basis of my lifestyle medicine practice and this book.

It is my mission to provide a roadmap to the simple, fact-based principles that offer us a lifetime of wellbeing and a path to your best health ever.

Your Best Health Ever!

THE CARDIOLOGIST'S SURPRISINGLY SIMPLE GUIDE TO WHAT REALLY WORKS

Your Roadmap To Natural Health

Are you healthy? Do you want to be healthy? Do we even know what being healthy means?

These seemingly simple questions are surprisingly difficult to answer.

As a cardiologist and practicing physician for over 15 years, I've seen thousands of patients, most of whom couldn't easily answer these questions.

Yet almost universally, we want to feel better, have more energy, reduce our risk of chronic diseases, and enjoy our time with our loved ones more.

On the surface, those goals don't seem so difficult. Yet in our society, they can often seem impossible.

I'm here to tell you that being healthy is a very achievable goal. The path to reaching that goal is an intricate mix of knowledge, motivation, and resilience, all of which I hope to share with you.

Close your eyes (I know it's hard to do when reading, but figuratively close your eyes) and picture that classic movie scene: someone running through a flowery meadow on a warm, sunny day, without a care, light on her feet, gentle breezes and the fragrance of spring in the air.

Now imagine that person is you, running lightly through the flowers, smiling and enjoying the sun as you go.

Open your eyes. What did you look like? What did your body look like? How much would you guess you weighed? How did your bones, joints and muscles feel as you ran through the meadow?

I bet you were smiling and your body felt light and strong, moving effortlessly and smoothly as you ran through the light crisp spring air. I bet you felt energetic, healthy, and perfectly happy to be you.

 Why are you not that person in real life? It's not that you don't want to be that person, or that you don't dream about being that person. Yet something is standing in your way, preventing you from becoming that person.

That's what I want to explore with you in this book. How do we identify the roadblocks that keep us from being the healthier, nimbler version of ourselves, and how do we overcome those obstacles and set our lives on the path to health?

A PILL-BASED SOCIETY

Unfortunately, our traditional healthcare model has evolved over time to focus more on managing disease instead of promoting health. A perfect storm of insurance payment models, overworked physicians, pharmaceutical company influences and government regulations has brought us to our current state.

High blood pressure? We have a pill for that. High cholesterol? Here's your prescription. Overweight? Not only do we have pills for that—we also have surgeries! We can induce medical bulimia by installing a valve in your stomach that empties the food you just ate. I didn't make that up. I wish I did.

Our society has become dependent on quick fixes, easy answers to make us appear healthier. Even worse, our government endorses this "quick fix" attitude by paying doctors more for making the numbers look good. Not for improving health, but for making the numbers look good. The assumption is that they are one and the same.

The truth is that taking pills to make our numbers look better is not the answer to feeling better and being healthier. Instead, that is the path to medication dependence and worsening overall health.

Each year thousands of people on cholesterol medications, blood pressure medications, and diabetes medications still experience life-threatening heart attacks, strokes and heart failure.

These medicines are not the cure-all we are frequently led to believe. In fact, they rarely cure anything. They're good at managing a symptom or improving a blood test, but they do little to address the underlying cause of the problem.

It doesn't have to be this way.

Scientific studies have shown that 60 to 80 percent of heart attacks are preventable with lifestyle interventions.

I will say that again.

Between 60 and 80% of heart attacks can be prevented!

Not with medication, but with real, meaningful, life changes.

You can take charge of your health. You can reduce your risk for diabetes. You can reduce your risk for heart disease, for strokes and for cancer. You can feel better and have more energy in the process.

Come with me on this journey as I show you how.

MY STORY

When I completed my general and preventive cardiology fellowship at Scripps Clinic and the Scripps Center for Integrative Medicine, I was full of hope about the power of health promotion and disease prevention.

As I transitioned into general practice, I was in awe of the incredible lifesaving tools we possessed as cardiologists: opening blocked arteries, replacing diseased heart valves, and correcting congestive heart failure.

Yet over time I grew frustrated as I saw how little effort we devoted to preventing the need for these procedures in the first place.

We would celebrate our success as we opened a patient's clogged artery. Then we would celebrate our success again, when we opened another blockage in the same patient.

Almost like clockwork, I'd soon see them return to the hospital for another stent, having a toe amputated due to diabetes, or drowning in their own body with congestive heart failure.

I started to ask myself, "Is this really a success? Wouldn't it be much more powerful if we could prevent the blockage in the first place?"

I started talking with my patients about how they lived, how they ate, how they exercised and how they managed their stress.

A consistent theme emerged. Most of them paid no attention to these aspects of their lives. They knew in a general way that nutrition and exercise could probably benefit their health.

Yet they had no concept of the powerful health benefits that lifestyle can provide.

Plus, they were on medications to take care of everything, right?

Add that to the contradictory recommendations circulating about lifestyle interventions, and it's no wonder they didn't know where to start.

I decided to take a stand, to try my best to reverse this trend in any way I could.

But here's my secret. I'm not interested in sensational sound bites or attention-grabbing headlines. I'm not going to try to wow you with extremes. We already have too many of those.

My quest is to serve as an objective and caring voice, to emphasize the importance of lifestyle and health promotion. I want to offer a reasonable analysis of how we can use lifestyle as medicine, and I want to show you how this helps you live healthier and live better. I hope to help more people than I can see in person or touch with my stethoscope, to show people how surprisingly simple it can be to improve your health.

If one person is able to improve their health and their life because of this book, it's all worth it.

....

Patients or Clients?

What term should we use to refer to those we are helping with their health? Patients? Clients? Health partners? To me, the word "patient" implies you are sick and need medical help. I see "patients" in the hospital on a regular basis. The patients I take care of are wearing dehumanizing hospital gowns, waked up every few hours to be poked and prodded by well-meaning hospital staff, and generally have life-threatening illnesses that need constant attention.

To be honest, I still don't know the best term for those whom I see in my office. We're working together to maintain their health and prevent disease. I think of them as "clients." I like the word client specifically because it doesn't sound medical. Even though I'm a medical doctor, I'm encouraging lifestyle as medicine, and don't want to associate it with sickness and disease.

One of my friends uses the term "health partner." I like the feel of this term, too. It suggests that we're a team, working to improve your health and vitality.

....

HEALTH VS WEIGHT

This book is not a weight loss book or a diet book. It is not a sensationalist book built around extreme ideas or extreme programs.

If you follow the tenets in this book, you will become healthier. You will reduce your risk of chronic diseases. Period.

Unfortunately, many people are more concerned about weight loss than they are about overall health. TV shows like "The Biggest Loser" and numerous commercial weight loss programs imply that weight loss and health are synonymous. They most definitely are not.

In fact, a study done on "Biggest Loser" participants showed that almost all of them fared poorly after the show was over. They experienced rapid weight gain with no improvement in their health.

Scientific studies have shown that technically overweight individuals who meet criteria for being "fit" have similar health benefits as those who are "normal weight."

In addition, skinny but sedentary people had worse health outcomes than fit overweight individuals.

Health is about much more than weight. When we can transform our lives and prioritize our health, appropriate weight loss will follow.

That's why I don't recommend using a scale as your guide to your success. Many of my clients are uncomfortable when I tell them to put their scale away for the next four weeks. They ask: "How will I know if the program is working? How will I know how I'm doing?"

You'll feel better, have more energy, and see the world in a brighter light.

Your pants will be a little looser.

You'll notice your exercise routine is getting easier and more comfortable.

You'll enjoy your meals, and you'll enjoy being mindful and being present.

And after four weeks, you'll also notice a positive impact on your blood work, your blood pressure, and other health markers.

Doesn't that sound better than just seeing a smaller number on a scale? It sure does to me. By the time you're done with this book, I hope it sounds better to you, too.

• •

A True Story

I saw a 45 year-old mother of three whose primary doctor had told her to start a statin to treat high cholesterol. Key facts:

- ⊙ Lab results: LDL 192, HDL 63, triglycerides 75
- ⊙ She exercised 6 days per week
- ⊙ She followed a low-fat diet
- ⊙ No other risk factors for cardiovascular disease
- ⊙ No family history of high cholesterol.

Very active, with no symptoms of heart disease, she was not at immediate risk, so we had time to evaluate her best path. We began with a thorough 20-minute discussion of statin benefits, risks and alternatives.

Based on this discussion, we decided to substitute lifestyle improvements for the recommended lifelong statin prescription. We altered her exercise, mixing more high-intensity training with moderate-intensity days and two "off days" when she walked her dog for an hour. We also improved her diet, adding healthy fats, increasing veggies and limiting sugars and simple carbohydrates. Finally, we added a couple of simple supplements.

Within four months, her inflammatory markers had all returned to normal levels. Her LDL had dropped to 125, HDL was up to 71, and her triglycerides were down to 63. Nine months later, her LDL was down to 99!

She achieved impressive results without a statin— and did so while increasing her fat intake!

Not everyone will see results like these. Some may still need prescription medications. For many, however, it makes sense to rethink your healthcare and start with lifestyle changes as your primary medicine.

....

THE PLAN

This book provides you with a simple four-week program built around the six building blocks of health. As you move through each step, you'll regain control of your health, feel better, and take another step on your path to your best health ever.

And because bumps in the road are inevitable, you'll also find a tune-up checklist and a troubleshooting guide in the Resources section. We're human, after all. The more we're prepared for inevitable slip-ups, the better we can recover.

I thank you for taking the time to come on this journey with me and for prioritizing your health.

Together, we'll reach your goals. You will become the **you** that you are meant to be.

1: What is Health?

Health means different things to different people, and it's surprisingly difficult to come up with a useful yet universal definition.

I can, however, tell you what health should **not** mean. It should not mean simply the absence of disease. Unfortunately, that is exactly how we tend to define it, in our society and in our medical community.

If you wake up on Monday without a diagnosis of Type 2 diabetes, on Monday we deem you "healthy."

If you go to the doctor on Tuesday and receive a diagnosis of diabetes, we now deem you as "no longer healthy."

Did the change really take place between Monday and Tuesday, while you were sleeping?

Of course not. You didn't just wake up one day with diabetes. It slowly emerged as a result of lifestyle choices which triggered a genetic predisposition.

The same holds true for heart disease, strokes, high blood pressure, dementia and many other chronic illnesses. The groundwork is laid for those diseases long before they are ultimately diagnosed.

If health is more than the absence of disease, what else is it?

I believe it's living a life in which you're happy, have the energy for the things you want to do, and see the world in a more positive light—while reducing your risk for developing chronic diseases in the future.

Based on my fifteen-year practice as a preventive cardiologist, I believe we have three distinct health dilemmas—our society's dilemma, our healthcare industry's dilemma, and our individual dilemma. These combine to keep us from living the life we want: a life full of energy and joy. In short, a life of *health*!

OUR SOCIETY'S HEALTH DILEMMA

Our country faces an overweight and obesity epidemic in adults, adolescents and children. Adult obesity increased from 22% in 1994 to 34% by 2012. Adolescent obesity increased from 12% in 2000 to 27% by 2014. The incidence of Type 2 diabetes and most chronic diseases has followed the same trend.

Why is this happening? Pick your reason: a more sedentary society caused by the rise of technology, increased consumption of sugary high-carbohydrate foods promoted by poor nutritional guidelines, hormonal changes caused by increased stress and poor sleep habits, changes in how we grow food and raise livestock, and many, many more.

We need an effective intervention, now. Otherwise, we will perpetuate this cycle by raising generations of children who truly cannot recognize the difference between real health and the mere absence of visible disease. After all, if we don't lead by example, how can we expect them to learn what health truly means?

THE HEALTHCARE INDUSTRY'S DILEMMA

Our current healthcare industry—our hospitals, pharmaceutical companies, medical device makers and healthcare providers—has certainly not solved the obesity and chronic disease epidemic we face. In fact, it's partly responsible for the rise of these problems.

Our healthcare system has become reactive. We're very good at putting band-aids on diseases and symptoms in the form of prescription drugs. Far too often these drugs mask the symptoms, without truly reversing the underlying trigger.

We simply add one problem to another: we introduce short-term and long-term medication side effects, while allowing the underlying cause to continue unabated.

Why has this happened?

Insurance payment models have pressured doctors to spend less time with patients.

Multibillion-dollar pharmaceutical companies spend millions marketing drugs as quick fixes.

Government regulations have often been misleading and based on poor science. They've offered financial incentives when patients reach certain health benchmarks like LDL levels, blood pressure readings, or glucose levels, motivating doctors to get to those goals as fast as possible.

All of these factors, and more, devalue the real work of medicine: getting to the root cause of disease and eliminating it for good.

They also create astounding conflicts of interest. For example, the pharmaceutical industry has one goal: to make money for their shareholders.

Their goal is not making people healthier, not helping you lead a happier life, not helping you exercise and eat right. Their business model depends on your *not* being healthy, and on your requiring their products.

Drug companies sponsor thousands of scientific trials every year, and they design those trials specifically to maximize the chances of scientific success for their drug.

Then they promote those trials to the public and to physicians, to convince all of us that we'd be far better off if we took their drug.

That's OK, you might think. Physicians should be able to see through the often-misleading marketing and set us on the best path, right?

Unfortunately, it's not that easy.

The average office visit is only 15 minutes. At least half of that is used for documentation.

Little time remains for your doctor to properly educate you about healthy lifestyle choices, motivate you to implement these choices, and thoroughly discuss the benefits, alternatives and risks of prescription drugs.

Those valuable, in-depth discussions will only become the standard when our system dramatically changes.

Fortunately, there is hope on the horizon.

New practice models, like concierge medical services, are emerging.

Important new specialties like functional medicine are also emerging. Functional medicine is a specific philosophy that places a greater emphasis on discovering the underlying causes of diseases, eliminating those causes, and restoring optimal health. This directly contradicts the too-common practice of putting a band-aid on symptoms by writing a prescription, while the underlying condition goes untreated.

I'm astounded, frankly, that this structure isn't taught in medical school. It seems so obvious. It is the best model for individual health.

....

Functional Medicine: Treating the Whole Person

A client asked me to help reduce her cardiovascular risk without the traditional prescription medications recommended by her physician. She had elevated cholesterol and inflammation markers, but the most glaring aspect of her evaluation was that significant hip pain limited her ability to walk and exercise. She loved being active, and was increasingly depressed by the forced reduction in her activity.

She had undergone routine x-rays and MRIs of her

hip. They did not identify any specific problems, and she had not found any help for her pain.

To help reduce her cardiovascular risk, we started her on a nutritional program. However, it was clear her physical and mental health depended on addressing her hip pain so she could get back to her activities.

We began by focusing on her posture, core strength, and other supporting structures for her hip. Before she knew it, her pain was gone and she was back to her regular exercise. Her outlook, nutrition and stress levels all improved—and of course, so did her cardiovascular risk!

• •

Why did this approach work? It treated her as a whole person, not just a collection of lab results and risk factors. Far too often providers see their piece of the puzzle—her hip, her diet, her cholesterol numbers—yet miss the big picture of how everything's related.

Don't get me wrong. Healthcare is not all "broken." We still need the amazing and miraculous tools and treatments that medicine offers, like emergency trauma surgery, heart angioplasty and stents to stop heart attacks as they occur, powerful antibiotics to treat life-threatening infections, insulin injections for Type I diabetics, life-saving surgery for cancer, and more.

But drugs and surgery are not the best answer for the chronic illnesses like diabetes and heart disease that plague our society. Investing the time to restructure our lifestyles and eliminate the root causes of these conditions will pay the greatest health dividend for ourselves and our society as a whole. That is the message the healthcare industry needs to champion.

As a society, we must demand this change, and make our voices heard by choosing healthcare providers who are committed to identifying and reversing the underlying causes of chronic disease through purposeful lifestyle changes.

As our collective voice grows louder, insurance providers and governmental regulating bodies will have to listen.

THE INDIVIDUAL HEALTH DILEMMA

What's most important is how we, as individuals, overcome these societal and industry health dilemmas.

What challenges do we face as we try to navigate through these systems?

How can we break through these barriers to achieve success with a healthy lifestyle?

I have seen it time and time again. Our lives are busy. We prioritize work, family, and social obligations. Time gets short, and our health goes to the bottom of the to-do list.

For example, eating well may require extra preparation and planning, taking extra time that we feel we don't have. The same holds true for finding the time and motivation to go for a walk or go to the gym.

Throw in vast amounts of contradictory health information, and it's no wonder health isn't a priority. Indeed, it seems less stressful to just let it slide.

Unfortunately, this very shortsighted approach puts us at risk down the road. Our mental and physical wellbeing, our happiness, and our lives all suffer when we don't prioritize our health.

Sometimes we tell ourselves that our health will become the priority "once I have a little more time," but in truth our risk of chronic disease and illness adds up during each minute we de-prioritize our wellbeing.

As individuals, therefore, our challenges are to:

- ⊙ Prioritize our health every day
- ⊙ Educate ourselves about what is truly healthy for us
- ⊙ Motivate ourselves to get started and take meaningful action
- ⊙ Maintain the path for a lifetime of health.

This guide will show you how to succeed at each of these challenges.

YOUR OPPORTUNITY

Understanding these challenges gives us a roadmap past the obstacles.

With the right tools, education, and a change in mindset, we can revolutionize our healthcare. We can demand true health promotion instead of a single-minded focus on "sick care" or "disease care."

We can refocus on our daily lifestyle and its crucial impact on our health, using our doctors as partners in knowledge rather than looking for a quick fix from a prescription.

As we make purposeful lifestyle changes to improve our health, we become grassroots motivators who help change the way our healthcare industry thinks and acts. We become living examples of the undeniable benefits of lifestyle changes—benefits that eliminate the root causes of chronic disease and promote health every single day.

As you turn to the next chapter, you're taking the first step on a journey to take charge of your health and make it your priority. You'll begin making real and meaningful changes that set you on a lifelong path to wellbeing.

Let's get started!

For journal citations and insights into the research discussed in this chapter, visit the Book Resources Blog at DrBretScher.com.

2: Using Science to Make Health Decisions

How do we know that a drug, or a lifestyle change like more exercise, helps our health? How do we know that poor stress reactions or lack of sleep harm our health?

Through scientific research. In fact, throughout this book I'll tell you about important scientific studies that form the basis for my recommendations. I'll explain the strengths and weaknesses of the study design, and share the key findings.

It's imperative that each of us knows how to interpret the research studies presented by the media and our healthcare providers.

Of course, that's easier said than done.

For starters, people without a strong science education are probably unfamiliar with the different types of scientific studies and their relative strengths and weaknesses.

In addition, most of us get our science news from unscientific sources like Twitter, Facebook, popular news reports, or even sensationalistic TV shows.

We quickly feel lost in a sea of contradictory advice, confused about which of the catchy headlines to believe.

The first step to taking charge of your health is to have the background knowledge to put the science into context and interpret for yourself what's probably worthwhile and what's more of a headline than a meaningful health tip.

I admit this can get a little dry, but that doesn't diminish its importance. This insight empowers you to decide what you can and cannot trust.

If you have a hard time making it through this chapter, skip it for now. Come back to it when we start discussing specific studies later in the book.

RETROSPECTIVE VS PROSPECTIVE STUDIES

A retrospective study looks back in time at events that have already taken place.

For instance, a retrospective study might look at the incidence of obesity and Type 2 diabetes that occurred following official dietary recommendations to eat less fat. The investigators would look at old records to define the scope of the problem before the recommendations were made, and then look again after the recommendations were implemented.

The study would likely conclude that the move towards eating low-fat foods was associated, or correlated, with increased obesity and diabetes.

This kind of study can never prove cause and effect. It can, however, demonstrate an association between several factors. It's generally the weakest level of evidence, but when you're examining historical data, it's the only choice available.

Prospective studies, on the other hand, start in the present day and collect evidence moving forward.

Say we changed the dietary guidelines today to limit sugar and carbohydrates and promote healthy fats. We would then track the incidence of obesity and diabetes over the next 10 years.

This kind of study still can't prove cause and effect. There could be many other changes that occur in that time frame, so-called co-variables. Despite this, it's still a stronger level of evidence than simply analyzing data from the past.

OBSERVATIONAL VS RANDOMIZED STUDIES

In observational studies, researchers simply observe the changes during a period without intervening. The retrospective and prospective studies described above are both observational studies.

An observational study of Whole Foods shoppers and McDonald's customers might tell us that Whole Foods shoppers have a lower risk of diabetes and heart disease.

But it wouldn't tell us why. The obvious thought would be that Whole Foods shoppers ate healthier foods. However, what if Whole Foods shoppers were less likely to smoke, more likely to exercise, or financially better off? Any of those factors could make them healthier—which would mean that Whole Foods itself wasn't completely responsible for the difference.

A randomized study would better account for those factors.

We could take 100 people who were as similar to each other as possible. They exercised the same, they didn't smoke, they had the same socioeconomic status, etc. We then randomly assign 50 of them to eat at Whole Foods and 50 to eat at McDonald's.

Since we chose where they eat, we eliminated the main variable of self-selection. Since we made sure they were similar to each other, we reduce the number of co-variables. The only remaining difference is our researchers' intervention: we told them where they could eat.

As you can see, the randomized study is a much stronger level of evidence than the observational study. It's much better at identifying the one intervention that affected the study's results.

CONTROLLED VS UNCONTROLLED STUDIES

In our McDonald's vs. Whole Foods example, we still haven't controlled for *what* they ate, only where they ate it.

You can get pizza at Whole Foods, or you could get a kale salad with wild salmon. At McDonald's, you can get a burger, fries and shake, or you could get a salad with a burger patty and no bun.

More controlled studies provide more specific and meaningful insight. Comparing the pros and cons of burgers vs. kale salad is a completely different and much more meaningful study than simply analyzing where people ate.

SELECTION OF STUDY PARTICIPANTS

It's always important to know who was included in a study.

Some studies are done on rats or mice or other members of the Animal Kingdom, yet the results are promoted as if they definitively apply to humans!

If a study were done on a uniform group of people in an isolated geographical area, would it still apply to you? Your genetics are different and your environment is likely very different.

Those differences don't make the results completely inapplicable. They do mean, however, that you should closely examine the relevance that the study may have to you as a unique individual.

META-ANALYSIS: STUDIES OF STUDIES

"Meta-analysis" studies combine multiple previous studies on a particular subject.

Say ten different studies compared eating at Whole Foods and McDonald's—but each study only had 10 to 20 participants. These sample sizes are likely too small to produce statistically significant conclusions. As studies get smaller, it's harder to prove a causative, or cause-and-effect relationship as opposed to simple chance.

However, if you combine these studies, you now have a group of almost 200 participants. The larger group size makes it easier to reach a conclusion with statistical certainty.

When looking at findings from a meta-analysis, the key is to understand which previous studies the authors decided to include or exclude from analysis, and why.

For example, say you included all studies that looked at vegetarian diets and the risk of diabetes. Depending on how many carbs and sugars participants ate, you might see what appears to be an increased risk of diabetes when people follow vegetarian diets.

But if you only included studies that looked at low-sugar vegetarian diets, you'd likely draw a very different conclusion.

Alternatively, if you included studies from the 1950s of vegetarian diets, those diets would be very different from today's vegetarian diets. Any conclusions you drew based on the combination of recent studies and older studies would likely not apply to modern society.

The bottom line: when reading about a meta-analysis, pay careful attention to how researchers chose the studies they included, and how that choice likely affected their conclusions.

ABSOLUTE VS RELATIVE RESULTS

News media outlets almost always report the *relative* risk reduction for a given drug or intervention. Why? It's more dramatic. It sounds more profound.

Here's a math question for a fifth-grader. If a drug reduces your risk of a heart attack from 1% over 5 years to 0.5% over 5 years, what is the risk reduction over 5 years? Easy, right? 1.0-0.5=0.5. The *absolute* risk reduction is half of one percent.

A news agency would report that as "An Incredible 50% Reduction!"

Technically, that's true, but that is the relative reduction; 0.5 is 50% of 1.0. The same could be said for a drug that reduces your risk of a heart attack from 50% to 25%. That also has a relative risk reduction of 50%; 25 is 50% of 50. But in this case the absolute reduction is 25%; 50-25=25.

Which number sounds more pertinent to you when deciding if you should take the medicine or undergo the intervention?

To me, it's clear that the absolute reduction is what I want to know. If all I know is the relative reduction, I have no idea what that means for reducing my risk.

When you read a sensational news story about an incredible benefit, make sure you clarify whether they're talking about a relative reduction or an absolute reduction. It makes all the difference.

THE NUMBER NEEDED TO TREAT

Hang in there with me while I get a little more technical. I want to briefly talk about the Number Needed to Treat (NNT). NNT is a number that represents how many people you need to treat to help one person. To calculate NNT, divide 1 by the absolute risk reduction.

For example, if a certain drug reduces absolute heart attack risk by 50%, represented in the equation as 0.5, then the NNT is 1/0.5=2.

This makes sense. You treat 2 people. 50% of those treated will benefit. You only have to treat two people to benefit one.

Here's a real-life example. Most primary prevention statin trials show a range of 0.5-1.6% benefit over 5 years. That equates to an NNT as high as 200 (1/.005) and as low as 62 (1/.016).

In other words, you need to treat between 62 and 142 people over 5 years to prevent an initial heart attack.

That puts the value of statins in a different light, doesn't it?

Remember the NNT when you read a story about a drug's benefit, or when your doctor prescribes a new drug.

It's eye-opening to realize how small the potential benefits sometimes are.

SENSIBLE SKEPTICISM

The best level of evidence is the prospective, randomized, controlled study. These studies are best at showing cause and effect.

The weakest evidence comes from the retrospective observational study.

These can point out an observed association, but can only rarely show cause and effect.

Meta-analysis studies combine other studies. Their strength is therefore dependent on the included trials. Some may be strong and others may be suspect.

Regardless of the type of study, be wary of dramatic conclusions promoted on TV and social media.

Remember the old saying among reporters: "If it bleeds, it leads."

Shocking headlines always get more attention—and after all, that's the media's primary goal.

The truth is rarely as exciting as the headlines.

———————

For further insight into NNT and other important ways you can use science to make smarter health decisions, visit the Book Resources Blog at DrBretScher.com.

———————

3: Your Mindset Is The Key

Here's the most important advice contained in this book: reframing your mindset is the number one step you can take to improve your health.

I commonly see clients who say, "OK, Doc. Tell me what to eat and how to exercise, and get me healthy." I appreciate the enthusiasm, but I know that all the knowledge in the world won't convince someone to live a healthy lifestyle if they don't have the proper mindset.

We need to *believe* that we can make the changes needed to be healthy, and we need to know that we can succeed.

With that belief, we can transform our lives. Without it, all the knowledge in the world is not enough.

I've seen countless clients who were labeled as having "failed lifestyle changes." They saw doctors for diabetes, high blood pressure, high cholesterol or other issues who instructed them to improve their nutrition and exercise.

Six months later, when nothing had changed, their doctors started them on medications.

By the time they see me, they already believe that lifestyle changes will never work for them. They believe that they simply cannot maintain meaningful changes that will make difference in their lives. They "failed lifestyle changes."

In reality, they already have some of the knowledge they need—but with a mindset that presupposes failure with no possibility of improvement, it's no wonder that they've been unable to make meaningful changes.

Our first step is almost always to work on reframing their mindset. Once they're educated about how to do this and have started on the right path, making the needed lifestyle changes suddenly becomes much more doable.

Consciously reframe your mindset, and change will begin to happen.

FIXED AND GROWTH MINDSETS

What does "mindset" even mean?

The most general definition is "a person's way of thinking and their opinions." It's a fixed attitude that predetermines how we interpret situations and react.

That term "fixed" implies that your mindset is set in stone, and cannot be changed. When we believe that's true, our mindset actually works against us. It prevents us from accomplishing our goals, health-related or otherwise.

Dr. Carol Dweck, a psychology professor at Stanford University, wrote the defining book about mindset, appropriately called *Mindset: The New Psychology of Success.*

Her main assertion is that we have two core mindset options: fixed and growth.

People with a fixed mindset tend to believe they have individual traits that are innate and cannot be changed or developed. These people tend to work in absolutes and avoid risks and challenges, because they find failure unacceptable and something that has to be avoided.

On the other hand, individuals with a growth mindset understand that their views and perceptions can change. They seek out challenges and see failure as a learning and growth opportunity. They don't get caught up with feeling inadequate. Instead, they look to constantly improve themselves, focusing on the process and not just the short-term results.

Dr. Dweck uses the concepts of fixed and growth mindsets to examine success and failure in business, sports, relationships, and even parenting.

I believe we should take the concept one step farther, and apply it to our health.

The Negative Feedback Loop

I'm sure you've experienced days when you're filled with energy, the sun is shining, the birds are chirping, and all seems right with the world. On those days, you tend to be more active, make better nutritional choices, and manage your stress better.

On the other hand, some days your body's aching and you feel fatigued and depressed. It seems like an insurmountable challenge to be active or to devote the time and mental energy to choose foods wisely. We may end up eating more sugary, high-carb "comfort foods," which in turn reinforces our fatigue and depression and leads to even more poor choices.

Before you know it, you're on medications for insomnia, depression, high blood pressure and Type 2 diabetes. Now, you're trying to deal with medication side effects in addition to your negative feelings. Eventually you feel like you've lost control of your health and your life.

Sounds awful, doesn't it? Just writing it is a little depressing. I wish I could say this is a rare occurrence, but I see it far too often in my cardiology practice.

This is the negative feedback loop that can hijack our attempts at a healthy life.

Sometimes people recognize the cycle they are in and are able to break out of it. More often, they don't even realize it. That is a dangerous situation, made even more dangerous if we feel that we cannot change.

STOP THE NEGATIVE FEEDBACK LOOP

When you're in a negative feedback loop, the most important intervention is to break the cycle. More knowledge about nutrition or exercise is always a good thing, but it won't get you out of this loop.

You need to alter your mindset to get you out of the loop. You need to reawaken your sense of purpose and your drive to be healthy.

I don't want to imply that this is always easy. Important and meaningful changes in life are rarely easy.

But with the right guidance and habits, these changes are very achievable.

REFRAME YOUR THOUGHT PROCESS

What if you could reframe your thought process so that you saw that things can and will get better?

What if you could gain control of your health and your life?

I have good news for you.

The truth is that you *can* reverse the negative cycle, you can start feeling better, you *can* start making better choices, and you *can* take control of your health.

Here's how you can start:

Define your goals in writing

Begin by defining your goals. Then, whatever your goals are, write them down.

Lose 30 pounds? Run a 10K? Reduce your heart disease or diabetes risk without drugs? Reduce your aches and pains and have more energy?

After you write down your goals, think about *why* you want to accomplish them.

Now write down those reasons.

Do you want to feel better so you can be more active with your kids, grandkids, or spouse? Do you want to have more energy to get through your workday, or feel better on the golf course? Write it down.

Do you want to lose weight so you can get rid of your chronic knee pain and feel better about yourself and your future? Or do you want to see a different person when you look in the mirror? Write it down.

Now, sign and date the paper. That makes it real and makes it yours.

Finally, put the paper somewhere safe and private, where you can easily retrieve it. Focusing on your goals is an excellent first step in paving your path to health.

Visualize what success will look like

This step is one of my favorite activities.

I want you to *visualize* how your life will look when you reach your goals.

Visualizing your accomplishments and feeling the emotions involved make it more real. Goals that feel more real are more obtainable.

Professional athletes, executives, motivational speakers and many other famous, and not-so-famous, people practice visualization to improve their performance.

I grew up as a swimmer, and I was fascinated by watching the Olympic swimmers before a race. Many of them would sit with their eyes closed, breathing quietly, visualizing the entire race in their mind. Hearing the starter's gun. Feeling the water as they dive in. Counting their strokes as they powerfully glide through the water. Feeling the emotion of touching the wall and looking up to see that they've just won the gold medal.

Visualizing their accomplishments from beginning to end attached that feeling of success to them, making it that much more real and achievable.

The same applies to any goal, including your health!

Sit down in a comfortable and quiet place. Close your eyes and visualize what it will feel like to accomplish your goals.

- ⊙ What will you look like?
- ⊙ How will you feel?
- ⊙ How much energy will you have?
- ⊙ How positive will your mood and outlook be?
- ⊙ How will your interactions with people be different?

Feels pretty good, doesn't it?

Now, go one step further.

Picture the new habits you've developed that help you maintain that goal.

- ⊙ What sleep habits do you have?
- ⊙ How about your exercise and physical activity habits?
- ⊙ How has your eating changed?
- ⊙ How do you react to stress?

This step is actually the most important one. Change doesn't just happen. It requires work. You have to change your daily habits in order to reach your goals. Visualizing those habits shows you your roadmap to accomplish your goals.

Many of us have set goals before, from New Year's resolutions to weight loss goals, stop-smoking promises, and more.

But I would venture to say that few of us have actually visualized accomplishing those goals, felt the emotion associated with achieving our goals, and even more importantly, visualized how our daily habits changed to support those goals.

When we see change as a magic black box that just happens, it forever remains a mystery. If we take the time to think about and visualize how our habits will change as we work towards our goals, we're arming ourselves with a roadmap to success.

From start to finish, your entire visualization exercise should only take 2-3 minutes. It's such a powerful tool to keep you focused on your goal that you should do it every day.

That's right, every day.

Since it only takes a few minutes, you can do it whenever it's convenient. The key is to just do it.

Ask "what-if" questions

Once you've defined your goals and visualized them, start asking positively-framed "What if" questions.

Studies show that 70% of our thoughts and questions are framed in a negative way. 70%! Those negative thoughts reflect a fixed mindset and an assumption that we are incapable of positive change.

- ⊙ "I probably won't be able to stick with a program and really accomplish all my goals."

- ⊙ "What if I mess up and fail?"

- ⊙ "Will everyone see me as a failure?"

If you think this way, your negative thoughts become self-fulfilling prophecies. Indeed, you fail— or worse, give up without even trying.

When you reframe your thoughts and questions to reflect a growth mindset—to embrace the possibility that you can change for the better—you increase the odds that you'll actually accomplish your goals.

- ⊙ "What if I *were* able to complete a program and get healthier and accomplish my goals?"

- ⊙ "What if I *am* able to feel better?"

- ⊙ "What if everyone sees how well I did and sees me as a success?"

You don't have to answer all the questions. Just asking them helps you start to reframe your mindset.

Reframing your "what if" questions sounds simple. And really, it is simple. But making it a habit does take some getting used to.

Since 70% of our daily thoughts are negative, positive thoughts may feel foreign and uncomfortable at first.

That's okay. Don't let that stop you. Keep asking the positively framed "what if" questions.

Like most habits, the more you do it, the more comfortable you'll become and the more likely it will become a longstanding personal habit.

Start the moment you wake up

Your best chance of having a positive mindset starts as soon as you wake up. From the moment you wake, embrace the day. Set the tone for the day that lies ahead by framing your mindset with a positive purpose.

Begin with a positive statement that sets your intention for the day, like "I deserve to be healthy, happy, and strong. I am grateful for what I have, and strive to be better."

Find a phrase that fits your personality, your goals and your purpose for the day.

Then, think about the day ahead. What's one specific thing you have to look forward to today? Maybe it's your lunch break at work, your morning walk, or the peace and quiet after the kids go to school.

Whatever it is, make it a positive thought and something to look forward to, and frame your day around that.

In the real world, we lead busy and stressful lives. We don't always wake up feeling refreshed and excited about the day to come.

Sometimes we're tired or groggy and we focus our attention on all the things we **have** to do and not the things we **want** to do.

Those negative feelings lend themselves to a fixed mindset that expects failure. Make a conscious effort to wake with a smile and set your positive intention for the day. You'll start to build the habit of positive thinking and a growth mindset that looks for opportunities rather than a fixed mindset that expects disappointment.

Did you know that even pretending to smile can change your brain chemistry?

That's right! Studies have shown that forcing a pretend smile can actually help us feel better.

So even if you don't feel like smiling, pretend you're biting down on a pencil. Your face will mimic a smile, and your brain may start to seem a little less congested, a little lighter, and a little brighter.

....

The Book of Awesome

I'm a big fan of Neil Pasricha's "The Book of Awesome."

He hit a rough patch in his life, and his outlook turned pretty negative. To break out of his negative feedback loop, he started writing down one thing that was "awesome" every single day.

The result was a wildly successful blog that became this book.

It sounds so simple, and yet it's very powerful. Why? It shows us how we can find something to be grateful for in almost anything.

Like peeling an orange in one shot. Sleeping in new bedsheets. When your suitcase is the first bag out of the luggage chute after a long flight.

I recommend that you get his book and read one

example every day when you wake up. It helps you frame your mindset to look for the "awesome" in your day.

You might just be surprised by where you find it!

••

Establish a daily ritual

Many behavioral psychologists emphasize the importance of physical daily reminders of your journey. They encourage us to develop our own "ritual of celebration" that we can do every day to remind us of our progress towards our goal. The ritual has two components—the act that reminds us of our progress, and the moment of celebration that accompanies it.

One of my clients decided that his tiny daily celebration—his reminder that he has the power to change for the better—would be a daily slow sit-up. Afterwards, he'd say, "This is my journey for health and happiness." Then, he'd do a little celebratory dance. After making sure no one else could possibly see him, of course.

He felt ridiculous at first, but he admitted that it felt good to celebrate. He worked out vigorously on a regular basis, but he didn't usually stop to appreciate the fact that he still prioritized taking care of himself even as his life had gotten more complicated and crunched for time.

Eventually, he included his kids in the ritual and celebration. Dancing around the living room celebrating with his kids was one of the most reaffirming actions he could imagine.

Celebrating our successes, no matter how small, is more than just a tremendous motivator. It can change the way our brains see the world and the way we experience our lives.

And after all, having a simple action every day that symbolically says "I am on this path to improving my health" does deserve celebration.

That simple action doesn't have to be complicated. For example, you could simply touch your reflection in the mirror and say, "This is the face of someone healthy."

Do it, say it, believe it—and celebrate it. High-five your partner or kids, do a five-second celebratory dance, or just shout "OOOOH YEAH!"

Pick what works for you, as long as it brings an emotional feeling of success.

Sound silly? You bet. It's the silly, unusual aspect of it that helps us break out of our loop and create new habits.

After all, you're celebrating more than just that simple action. You're celebrating the work in progress that is your life, your journey, and your health.

Find your purpose

In his book *Blue Zones*, Dan Buettner investigated the most common habits in societies where people frequently live into their 90s and 100s. One of the most important, called "ikigai" in Okinawa, Japan, was finding your purpose. The term "ikigai" basically translates to "why I wake up in the morning."

He hypothesizes that this sense of purpose allows the individuals to reduce their sense of stress. That certainly makes sense, and I would add that when you identify with a sense of purpose, you tend to like yourself better. You understand your importance, and thus you see the value in taking better care of yourself.

That is why I encourage you to find your purpose. You can pick a lifelong purpose as grand as finding the cure for cancer, or as close to your heart as spending time with your grandkids, and everywhere in between.

You can also choose a daily purpose. "Today my purpose is to be a supportive partner." "Tomorrow it will be to help teach someone to be generous."

Find your passion and make it your purpose— today, tomorrow and in the future. That way you'll respect yourself and want to take better care of yourself.

Design success into your day

Why is it that some people seem to have more will power than others?

It turns out that self-control and willpower are limited resources. We draw constantly on these resources throughout the day, so it's really no surprise that they wear thin by evening. We've been exerting our self-control and making good choices all day, and now, we're *done*!

In many cases, those who seem to have more willpower have simply orchestrated their day so that they use up fewer "willpower units." That way, when they need to call on their self-control, they still have plenty in the tank.

The most common time for many of us to "slip" or deviate from our healthy habits is at the end of the day when our willpower units have been depleted. We let our healthy routines lapse. We start making worse nutritional choices. We decide to sit on the couch rather than go for a walk.

The first action is to not beat yourself up over it. Understand it and acknowledge it, but do not punish or berate yourself over it.

The next step is to take positive action to help control these lapses in the future. If you can control your environment better, you won't need to rely on your self-control as much.

For example, if you find yourself unable to resist ice cream or cookies at the end of the day:

- ⊙ Make sure these treats aren't available. Don't buy them.

- ⊙ Explain to your family why it's important for you to keep these temptations out of the house. Many people don't want to admit that they have trouble with self-control. It seems weak or like a failure. Just the opposite! Understanding your limits is the key to success.

- ⊙ Share this chapter with them so that they better understand the limited nature of self-control.

- ⊙ Avoid hanging out in the kitchen where it's all too easy to grab snacks you don't need.

- ⊙ Read or spend time with family in a different room, or sit outside

- ⊙ Go for a walk or do 10 minutes of exercise. Getting your blood pumping and endorphins (brain and nervous system hormones) flowing helps you reset your self-control and make better decisions.

The key is changing your environment to take self-control out of the equation. Create an environment that requires you to use your self-control units less often, and you'll see immediate improvement when you do need them.

Keep an accountability calendar

An accountability calendar helps you remember your week and spot opportunities to make better decisions in the future.

Simply write your goals at the top of the calendar page. Every day, jot a quick note summarizing your choices for the day.

"Did great eating out, researched the menu and made smart choices" or "Cheat day, had pizza and too many beers out with the guys."

That way you can accurately gauge your progress without relying on memory.

For example, if you scan your accountability calendar for the last week and see "Friday night birthday party, had 3 beers and 3 pieces of pizza," you might be less inclined to indulge when you have dinner with your spouse.

You might also spot a tendency to overeat at office potlucks, and decide that you'll start bringing your own lunch on those days. Or you may notice you make unhealthy snack choices during your day. That may motivate you to pack apples and nuts when you go to the office to keep you from dipping in to the office candy jar.

Your accountability calendar takes some of the pressure off, so you don't have to keep your self-control switched to "on" 24/7. Your calendar helps you plan better actions in the future that won't call on your willpower.

Surround yourself with the power of community

You don't have to go it alone. Many goals seem impossible when we tackle them by ourselves—yet they can become fully within reach when we work on them together.

Research has shown that people who feel a greater sense of community are happier, less depressed, and enjoy more meaningful interactions.

Who should be part of your community? Anyone who supports your commitment to your goals in a positive way. Tell trusted family members and close friends your goals. Gauge their responses and recruit those who respond in a way that will be honest yet supportive. You can even draw up a contract to make it "official." They now have this responsibility, as a member of your support community.

Your social media network can also be a great place to find like-minded people who'll support your journey to better health.

Ideally, your healthcare providers will also be part of your team. That means you need to share your goals and intentions with them, and actively recruit them into your community.

Our community is there to celebrate with us when we succeed and help pick us up when we fall. It can also help hold us more accountable than we'll hold ourselves.

Alone, it's easy to convince yourself that an extra martini or another cookie won't hurt. It's easy to convince yourself that sleeping late instead of exercising won't hurt. It's much tougher to convince our community members that those actions are acceptable.

....

Be Your Own Caddie

Don't worry, this isn't about golf. This is about being kind to yourself, encouraging yourself, and supporting yourself.

I'm not a very good golfer. Sometimes I'm downright awful, and I can get very frustrated. It's all too easy to say to myself, "How could you do that!" "That was so stupid!" "Are you kidding me with that shot? What's the matter with you?"

I'm not proud of that. No surprise, my next shot often just gets worse. How could I expect anything else with such a negative mindset?

Would a golfer's caddie ever say "You are an idiot! You are a terrible golfer! How could you hit such an awful shot?"

Of course not! But that doesn't stop us from saying that to ourselves.

3: YOUR MINDSET IS THE KEY

The same is true when it comes to a healthy lifestyle. It's all too easy to get down on ourselves. "How could I be such an idiot for eating that ice cream? I have no willpower, I'm too weak to resist!" "I'm such a lazy slug. I can't even get 8,000 steps in a day. What in the world is wrong with me?"

Be Your Own Health Caddie

When these thoughts creep in, ask yourself if your caddie would say those things to you. If not, reframe your thoughts the way your health caddie would say them:

"Sure, you shouldn't have had the whole carton of ice cream. What a great learning experience. Take note of how you feel at this moment and remember that next time you start to dig into the ice cream." "You got 6,000 steps today. That's certainly better than none. Let's find ways to get you to 8,000 tomorrow."

Doesn't that sound better?

Negative Thoughts Worked Well...For Cavemen

Behavioral researchers estimate that we have approximately 60,000 thoughts a day, 70% of which are negative. That's a whole lot of negativity. No wonder life sometimes seems so hard!

Millions of years ago, this might have served us well. When your primary goal is survival, you constantly think about threats and dangers. Is that a saber-tooth tiger? RUN! And your mind remembers that spot much more vividly than the beautiful flowers you saw earlier in the day.

When our goal is health and happiness, that negative bias that seeks out threat and danger works against us. It promotes a fixed mindset that

limits our ability to find creative solutions and
develop the skills needed to grow.

The Science of Positivity

What if we had our health caddie with us all the
time to transform our negative thoughts into
positive thoughts?

Brain imaging and blood testing has shown
that positive thoughts trigger a cascade of
brain activation and hormone release which
promotes relaxation and calm. Randomized
trials have shown that positive thoughts reduce
illness symptoms and increase mindfulness and
a feeling of purpose. That translates into better
overall health and greater success with lifestyle
programs.

Be Mindful and Play

Our health caddie would also encourage us to
practice regular mindful meditation, which studies
show increases daily positivity.

And our caddie would also remind us to play,
which increases positivity by stimulating the brain
in ways similar to meditation.

What's play? It's what you enjoy doing. That's
probably not 30 minutes on an elliptical trainer.
More likely, it's going dancing, playing mini-golf
with family or friends, or playing an intense game
of Monopoly.

Place Happiness Before Success

Most behavioral research suggests that success
follows happiness, not the other way around.
Said another way, success doesn't increase your
chances of being happy, but being happy does
increase your chances of success.

If you're a negative thinker, then achieving a

predefined goal probably won't change that. Focus on positive thinking, and you're much more likely to engage the world with a growth mindset and develop the skills and talents needed to succeed.

Let your own inner health caddie flourish!

••

CONCLUSION

Perfection is not the goal. *Finding a way to incorporate health into your life* is the goal. You need easily accessible tools to help you maintain healthy practices, break out of the inevitable negative feedback loop and reframe your life with a positive spin.

Here's the biggest tip of all: you will not be perfect, yet you *will* improve.

Never stop asking, "How can I improve upon this?" and "How can I make a better decision next time?"

Focus on a growth mindset. Imperfection is nothing more than a learning opportunity for growth and improvement. Challenges are just opportunities to find new ways to move forward on your path to health. Once you truly believe this, you are ready to succeed.

Visualize your goals and the habits needed to achieve them. Start your day with a purpose and a plan for success. Create the daily habits that help you see the world as an opportunity, and look for the "awesome" in every day.

Remember to celebrate your successes and your habits, and embrace your purpose.

Recognize your transgressions, accept them, and vow to be better. Be accountable but don't beat yourself up, get angry, or get down on yourself. Remind yourself that "I am the kind of person who can fall down, get right back up, and stay on target." Then make your plan to get even-by getting better!

Find your purpose, treat yourself kindly and with respect, and you'll be your own best partner in your quest for health and happiness.

THE PLAN: MODIFY YOUR MINDSET

Week 1

⊙ Define your goals, write them down and sign the paper. Take time to visualize what it looks like to accomplish those goals. Remember to visualize the habits that coincide with achieving those goals, too. Start asking your positively framed "What if" questions.

Week 2

⊙ Develop a personal statement that resonates with you and helps establish your path to healthy habits. Say this statement aloud when you wake up every day to help set your intention for the day. Along the same lines, search for both your short-term and long-term purpose.

Week 3

⊙ Add a simple daily action to remind you of your goals and your purpose. Perform this action every day and celebrate it. It doesn't count if you don't celebrate it!

Week 4

⊙ Start an accountability calendar. Review it on a weekly basis to celebrate your successes and spot opportunities for improvement.

———

For further insight into the growth mindset and Dr. Carol Dweck's research, visit the Book Resources Blog at DrBretScher.com.

———

4: Nourish Your Body

REDEFINING EATING

You will never hear me using the word "diet" to mean eating to lose weight. And you won't hear me describe eating as "fueling your body." This is not a crash diet book. It's a framework for regaining your health. Diets don't work long-term. They suggest restrictions and limitations. They suggest that one pattern of eating is right, and the others are wrong. That approach may produce some immediate improvements, but it is rarely sustainable.

Instead, I call eating what it should be: **nourishing your body**.

After all, the purpose of eating is to provide your body with the nourishment it needs, to provide energy, to eliminate hunger, and hopefully, to provide enjoyment.

When we start to look at food from this perspective, we gain a much clearer understanding about what it means to be healthy.

Everything we eat either helps or hurts our bodies. Does what you are about to eat provide you with nourishment, energy, enjoyment and eliminate your hunger? If not, just say "no" and look for an alternative that does.

It's just food, right? Why does it seem so complicated?

For better or for worse, food is a constant and essential presence in our lives. It's an integral part of our society, our social life, and our reward system. We therefore have a very intimate and complicated relationship with food.

So while that can make it harder to change our nutritional habits, it also makes it that much more important to address them.

There is no shortage of books, blogs, or videos telling you what to eat. Unfortunately, many of these directly contradict each other. In addition, everyone who promotes health through lifestyle and nutrition has a bias, me included. That makes it very difficult for any of us to know when we can truly trust specific recommendations. I hope this book will give you the tools to help you decipher when you can trust information, and when you should interpret it with skepticism.

Nutritional science is messy. It is nearly impossible to study just one aspect of food, and when we do, it is rarely practical to apply it to everyday life. After all, we don't eat "protein, with a side of fat and carbohydrate." We eat food!

For example, these two meals could both be categorized as "fish" or "protein." They'd look comparable in a food journal—but I guarantee you that they affect your body differently:

Meal 1	Meal 2
6-ounce wild Alaskan salmon filet baked in olive oil & lemon juice, served on a bed of cooked spinach and kale	Farmed cod fish tacos topped with special sauce, garnished with a few shreds of cabbage, served on flour tortillas

Moreover, research studies frequently rely on food journals, which require study participants to accurately remember and record exact amounts of food and all the ingredients. When you sit down to catch up on your food journal and try to remember what you ate the day before, you could easily categorize either of the above meals as "fish with vegetables."

See what I mean when I say nutritional science is messy?

Try it for yourself. Can *you* remember the details of everything you ate last week? How about yesterday?

It's not an easy task. You can see why there's no shortage of controversies about what the science really means.

So how can you know the "right" way to eat?

How can we separate real science from fiction?

THE EVIDENCE FOR NUTRITION

Nutritional science experiments are not only difficult to design, but can be even more difficult to interpret. In this section, I'll share real world examples of how we can interpret the science and, more importantly, how you can directly apply that to your everyday nutritional choices.

Let's start with the areas of broad agreement first.

Areas of scientific agreement

Eat real food

A shocking study in 2015 showed that Americans get 61% of their calories from moderately or heavily processed foods. Over half! That means over half of our food consumption contains hidden sugars, trans fats, cheap and refined oils, preservatives, additives, fillers, and other potentially harmful products.

In other words, 61% of our food isn't even food! Why would we do that?

Cost, convenience, and a multi-billion dollar food industry, that's why. But here's a secret that isn't really a secret: the food industry does not care about your health. They're businesses, just like any other. Their commitment is to their stockholders and their bottom line. Your health doesn't factor into that equation.

That's why we need to reframe how we choose the food we eat. We need to accept responsibility for what goes into our bodies. If food didn't come directly from the ground or from an animal, then we shouldn't eat it.

Eat food in its original form as much possible. Avoid fake food made in factories.

Simple as that.

My favorite is comparing fresh, from the earth vegetables to the popularized "vegetable chips."

Which one do you think has the most to offer your body?

Or fresh, raw tomatoes as opposed to tomato juice with all the beneficial fiber removed. Or even worse, pasta sauce with added sugar and preservatives. These aren't real foods, and we shouldn't think of them as real food.

The food you eat should not **have** ingredients, it should **be** its own ingredient.

Most commercial diets are initially successful because they reduce or eliminate the processed junk from our diets—items like cookies, cakes, doughnuts, crackers, muffins, and chips. These processed foods don't provide sustainable energy or adequate nutrition. Nor do they reduce hunger for more than a brief moment.

Since these foods lack nutrients and are packed with empty calories from sugar and refined carbohydrates, simply cutting them out of your diet will always improve your health and aid weight loss.

As a culture, we like to think we can improve everything with our vast knowledge of chemistry and our amazing technology. When it comes to our food, however, we can't do any better than Mother Nature. So let's stop trying, and let's get back to the basics of eating real food.

If that's the one and only change you make, you're well on your way to improving your health and reducing your risk of chronic diseases.

....

Simple Swaps

Eat more real food with these simple swaps! Instead of cereal, muffins or bagels for breakfast, throw leftover veggies and one or two eggs into a pan, add a slice of avocado and a sprinkle of Celtic sea salt. A delicious way to start your day, in less than five minutes!

Instead of manufactured snacks like chips, crackers, or cookies, snack on a couple handfuls of nuts. Try celery and carrot sticks dipped in hummus or nut butter.

For dessert, try a fruit salad with berries, apples, oranges and other naturally sweet fruits.

Your swaps don't have to be perfect. Any improvements you make will directly benefit your health. As you experiment, simple substitutions will become a healthy habit.

....

Eliminate added sugars

Despite arguments about which sugars are better (high fructose corn syrup vs. sucrose vs. maltose, etc.), the bottom line is that all sugars raise your blood glucose and insulin levels to varying degrees. They therefore contribute to fat storage, because insulin is a fat storage hormone. They also contribute to blood sugar-related diseases ranging from diabetes to heart disease, dementia, fatty liver and others.

It turns out that the source of sugar is the most important factor determining its health effects.

White sugar, high-fructose corn syrup, and other processed, refined sugars made in factories provide only quick, short-lived energy and have no nutrients. Without the fiber from real foods, your body quickly absorbs the refined sugar and starts a cascade of harmful effects, like quick blood sugar spikes and crashes, and a sustained rise in insulin.

These products also stimulate the dopamine reward centers in your brain in the same way as addictive drugs like cocaine.

That's right. Sugar is a drug. It acts like an addictive drug in your brain. Food companies know this all too well and they test their recipes on subjects to find the maximal stimulation of the brain's reward center. This ensures that you want more and more. As the old potato chip commercial said, "We bet you can't eat just one."

So in a way, it isn't completely your fault that you can't stop eating the sugary treat in front of you. Hundreds, perhaps thousands, of hours of research likely went into that treat to make sure that would happen.

On the other hand, sugar from a peach, or from berries, or from an apple acts differently in your body. Sugars from real food tend to be much less concentrated. They also come with the beneficial fiber and other nutrients that slow sugar absorption, and reduce blood sugar and insulin swings. In the brain, they reduce dopamine "reward center" activation. So even though naturally-occurring sugars have a similar chemical structure to manufactured sugars, they trigger a vastly different response from your body.

Scientists have also learned that our taste buds develop a tolerance to sugar. What was once too sweet can become just right. One spoonful of sugar in your coffee easily turns into two or three over time.

Think about this: We frequently add sugar, salt or fat, like butter, to our food to make it taste better. Would you ever eat a handful of salt by itself? No way. How about a whole stick of butter? Ugh. Of course not. So there appears to be a logical limit to how much we'll eat at one time.

But kids don't hesitate to suck down an entire pixie stick—made of nothing but pure sugar. There's no limit in sight when it comes to sugar. That's a definite problem because added sugar intake is related to chronic inflammation, obesity, diabetes, heart disease and premature death.

There is good news, however. We can train our taste buds to want less sugar as we taper our sugar consumption over time. And some healthcare providers believe that reducing added sugar is the best thing you can do for your health other than quitting smoking.

The advice is simple. Don't add sugar to your coffee or tea. Don't drink sugary fruit juices or dessert shakes masquerading as coffee drinks. Avoid baked goods, candy and processed foods with added sugars. Even if the package says "organic" or "natural," or even "gluten free," there is nothing natural about the concentrated sugar and its errant effects on our bodies. If you need to satisfy your sweet tooth, eat organic berries, melon, peaches and other natural fruits. Over time your taste buds will adjust and your health will improve!

Your best weapon for avoiding the numerous dangers of added sugar is to simply focus on real, minimally processed foods.

....

Everything In Moderation

I bet you've heard that healthy eating involves everything in moderation. The idea is that there are no inherently "good" foods or "bad" foods. It sounds like my kind of advice. Simple. Not overly restrictive. Friendly. The problem is that it may not actually work.

A 2015 observational study showed that those who ate with greater diversity and included more foods in moderation had a significantly larger waist than those who ate less varied foods. For these subjects, "everything in moderation" did not improve their health.

Why? We tend to alter our definition of moderation based on how much we typically eat, and how much we like the food in question. For most, a moderate amount of ice cream is larger than a moderate amount of Brussels sprouts. And the amount of ice cream we usually eat is likely to be our definition of moderate.

We've become accustomed to the oversized portions found in any Cheesecake Factory, Hometown Buffet, or old-fashioned American deli. Just looking at these inflated sizes would nauseate many people in Europe, Africa and Asia.

We're also forgetful. When Saturday rolls around and we "reward" ourselves with pizza, beer and a sundae, it is natural to forget about the pizza and ice cream we had with the kids Wednesday night. Or the birthday cake for our co-worker on

Tuesday. It becomes easy to feel we are still within "moderation."

It turns out that there really are good foods and bad foods. Vegetables are good. Added sugar is bad. I can't imagine ever suggesting drinking sugary sodas in moderation or eating a pure sugar pixie stick in moderation.

So where do we draw the line? Muffins? Bagels? Mocha Frappuccinos?

Some of us are simply better at controlling "moderation." For others, our brain's dopamine centers are too sensitive to reasonably limit the addictive properties of sugar and some other food choices.

If you're like this, you may be better off following the "all or none" approach. Avoid all sugar, avoid all alcohol, avoid all white flour and simple grains. That way you won't have to worry about controlling your cravings.

All things in moderation may work for some—but only in moderation!

....

Make your meals vegetable-based

Over the decades, one truth has held steady in the scientific literature: vegetable consumption is associated with better heath.

Vegetable intake has been associated with a decreased risk of cancer, heart disease, diabetes, hypertension, and more. Plus, eating a variety of colorful vegetables provides an array of beneficial phytonutrients, plant compounds that benefit overall health and prevent disease.

It is beyond argument at this time that veggies should be the basis of a healthy diet.

Eating vegetable-based meals isn't the same as being a vegetarian. Tofurky and tempeh are popular processed vegetarian staples, but they are not vegetables and have not been shown to have the same beneficial effects as real, from-the-earth vegetables.

Your first challenge is to reframe the way you see your plate. Fifty to seventy-five percent of each meal should consist of real vegetables. That is a major shift from current norms, where the main dish is a huge plate of pasta or a 16-ounce steak, and vegetables are relegated to a small side dish.

Choose mostly non-starchy vegetables like these:

- ⊙ Spinach
- ⊙ Kale
- ⊙ Chard
- ⊙ Broccoli
- ⊙ Cauliflower
- ⊙ Zucchini
- ⊙ Mushrooms
- ⊙ Onions
- ⊙ Asparagus
- ⊙ Tomatoes

Choose some, but fewer, starchy veggies like these:

- ⊙ Sweet potato
- ⊙ Butternut squash
- ⊙ Beets
- ⊙ Corn
- ⊙ Peas

You can start to see a pattern here. A real-food, vegetable-based diet without added sugars is clearly the way to go to improve your health and reduce your risk of cancer, diabetes, heart disease, neurocognitive diseases, and many other chronic illnesses.

TIP ⊙ People routinely underestimate the amount of vegetables they eat. In my experience, people also hate measuring cups of food and counting their servings. So we all need to get better at estimating how many vegetables we eat. Vegetable-based means just that. Find a great vegetarian cookbook that focuses on a variety of vegetables and minimally-processed foods. The Recommended Reading section lists some of my favorites. Make the recipes and then add your favorite protein and fat to the meal as a side dish.

Eat natural monounsaturated fats

Not all fats are created the same. The one fat that is beyond controversy is minimally processed monounsaturated fat, found in olive oil, avocados, nuts and seeds.

The Mediterranean diet, consisting of over 40% fat, primarily from monounsaturated fats, is the only primary nutritional intervention shown to reduce heart attacks and strokes.

The scientific literature clearly demonstrates that monounsaturated fats increase "good" HDL cholesterol, do not worsen and possibly improve "bad" LDL cholesterol, and likely reduce LDL-related inflammation. They provide nourishment, decrease hunger, reduce sugar and insulin spikes— and best of all, are enjoyable!

It is beyond controversy that we should add more nuts, avocado, olives and olive oil to our nutritional choices. That doesn't mean we should only choose those options when they happen to be convenient. It means actively seeking to increase our consumption of these foods. Look for ways to add them to every meal.

As always, these fats should come from naturally occurring, less processed real foods.

TIP ❯ Most salad dressings are full of added sugar and other processed ingredients. If you use olive oil as your salad dressing instead, you eliminate the stuff you don't want, and increase the nutrients that you do want! You can even use olive oil with a squeeze of lemon or lime to add to the taste.

Also, use almond oil or avocado oil as your main cooking oil to increase your healthy fat intake and exposure to monounsaturated fats.

Avoid manufactured trans fats

Manufactured, or industrial, trans-fats are used by food manufacturers to increase the shelf life of various processed foods including fried foods, pizza, microwave popcorn, cakes, cookies, pie crusts, crackers and other baked goods.

Research has shown that these fats increase the risk of cancer, cardiovascular disease, and other chronic health conditions. They increase your LDL while lowering your HDL, a particularly dangerous combination. Even worse, they increase the oxidation that leads to unstable cholesterol buildup in your arteries and cause greater inflammation throughout your body.

If you're eating only real foods, you're already avoiding industrial trans fats. That's because industrial trans fats are made in laboratories, not in nature. Food companies produce trans fats by chemically adding hydrogen to liquid oils.

Natural trans fats, on the other hand, are likely not harmful. They occur in the milk and meat from ruminant animals—those that graze on plants and grasses—like cows, sheep, elk, bison and others.

These fats consist mainly of conjugated linoleic acids, also known as "CLA." Studies have shown that CLA may actually be beneficial for our health, possibly reducing the risk of cancer and heart disease.

Fortunately, many food companies and restaurant chains are actively reducing their use of industrial trans fats. But that doesn't mean they are gone. We still need to be vigilant about reading the labels of our food to make sure it has zero trans-fats.

Remember, food is not innocuous. Everything we eat either helps us or hurts us. There is no question that industrial trans fats are harmful. Once again, just eat real food and you're already avoiding dangerous trans fats.

Eat the minimum calories needed

Aim for eating only the calories you need to maintain an active and enjoyable lifestyle.

Food is meant to nourish our bodies and provide energy. Once we've met those requirements, extra calories do nothing beneficial for us. Instead, they're directly associated with weight gain and blood glucose-related diseases.

I acknowledge that it can be difficult to know in the moment whether you're full, especially surrounded by our "supersize" and endless buffet culture.

These tips will help you learn what "full" really feels like:

- ⊙ Be mindful as you eat. Eating while distracted is an easy way to overeat without realizing it. Staying mindful keeps you more in tune with your body and helps you "check in" with your hungry/full balance.

- ⊙ The brain takes 20 minutes to realize that we're full. So it's best to underestimate how full you think you are and eat only until you're 75% full. Over time, you'll become more aware of how much you need to eat.

- ⊙ Avoid buffet-style eating, since this easily leads to over-eating. Serve yourself on a single plate and know that this is all you will eat.

- ⊙ Use smaller plates. This gives you a visual cue that you're eating enough, versus a large plate that's not completely filled.

- ⊙ Don't feel obliged to clear your plate. Many of us were told this as kids, and now we feel guilty about throwing away food.

TIP ⊙ To avoid guilt about food waste, start a compost bin!

The Worm Bin 360 and Worm Café are space-efficient ways to make use of your leftover food. The end-result is an incredible and guilt-free fertilizer for your plants and garden. Plus my kids love our worms! It's like they have 1000 new pets. Just don't ask me to remember all their names....

Alternatively, save your food scraps and donate them to a local farm. The Coastal Roots farm in San Diego, where I volunteer, is an excellent example. They use donated food scraps to feed their chickens. What a great idea!

Control your surroundings

We like to talk about "willpower" as if it were something we all should master and enjoy in unlimited amounts. We also talk about it as an all-or-none phenomenon—we either have it or we do not.

The truth, however, is much different.

Willpower is not an absolute. It is a skill that takes practice, patience, and persistence to build.

Like a muscle, it may strengthen over the long-term, but the more you use it, the more fatigued it gets in the short-term. And there is always a limit to how much willpower you have.

Say there's an unhealthy but tempting food choice nearby. When you're rested, patient and mindful, you may be able to avoid it 90% of the time using willpower.

That success rate will drop dramatically when you're more tired, more distracted, and less mindful. More often than not, that occurs at the end of the day.

It makes perfect sense, doesn't it? After a long day of work, dealing with multiple responsibilities and decisions, the last thing we want to do is be vigilant about more decisions. Instead, we want to relax and let our minds go. That's when our willpower is most likely to falter.

Faltering willpower is also related to the degree of temptation offered by a particular food.

We all have those treats that carry emotional weight with us. They bring back memories of comfort, joy, and pleasure. Unfortunately, those feelings quickly fade when we get the sugar high and sugar crash from the junk we just ate.

The best way to improve your chances of success in avoiding these pitfalls is to control your surroundings.

Make sure those "feel good" treats are simply not available to you at times when you find your willpower units are at their lowest.

If it isn't in your house or office, chances are, you're not going to eat it. That way you don't have to rely on your willpower all the time.

If you live by yourself and do all the shopping, you only need to convince yourself of this principle. It gets more complicated, however, when you have a spouse, children, or other family members sharing the same kitchen, refrigerator, and pantry.

That's when it becomes crucial to recruit your housemates into your community.

They need to understand your goals and the reason that you need to control your surroundings. Once you enroll them into your support community, it will be much easier to control your environment and still maintain a happy household.

Controlling your surroundings also applies to eating out, which can easily become the ultimate loss of control over what we eat.

Try these tips:

- ⊙ Scout out the menu ahead of time so you know what you're going to order and you know what substitutions or modifications you plan to request.

We've all experienced visiting an unfamiliar restaurant, getting wrapped up in the conversation—and all of a sudden, it's time to order.

We get a little rushed and end up picking the first thing we see that looks good, without giving it much thought. That's a very common way to lose control of your environment and end up eating things you would not have otherwise chosen.

- ⊙ See the menu as a suggestion, not a hard rule.

Remember, you're paying them for the food. They want you to be happy and come back. If you ask for a modification, like substituting a side salad for fries, or ordering a half-portion, they should be more than happy to accommodate you.

- ⊙ Limit sauces and salad dressings.

They often hide sugar and non-nourishing calories. Use olive oil instead!

- ⊙ Don't let dessert surprise you.

Eating out is fun, and dessert is frequently an integral part of that experience.

Anticipate this, and suggest ordering one dessert for the table to share as opposed to two or three. Never have the first bite, and never have the last bite. That will help minimize the damage.

Eat mindfully

We've all probably eaten an entire bowl of whatever was in front of us when we were watching television, using our computer or were otherwise distracted. In fact, science supports the claim that distracted eating leads to unhealthy overeating.

Whether it was something relatively healthy like a bowl of nuts, or something not so healthy, like cookies or a bag of chips, eating too much is bad for our health. And it's easy to do to when we're distracted.

Fortunately, the opposite is also true. If we're mindful when we eat, and stay fully present, we tend to eat less. We still eat what we need. We don't leave ourselves hungry. But we're able to avoid the mindless overconsumption of calories that our bodies don't need. Remember that I said earlier that it takes about 20 minutes for your brain to realize you're full. If you're distracted in that 20-minute period, you're likely to keep eating without even realizing it.

Mindful eating is very helpful for slowing down, appreciating your food, controlling your portions, and helping you realize when you're full. It's also an excellent opportunity to continue your lifelong practice of mindfulness.

No matter the situation, we will always benefit from the opportunity to be fully present, to experience our surroundings, to acknowledge our feelings, and to become better at recognition and control. Focus on the food you are eating, understand when you are no longer hungry, and stop before you're completely full.

These suggestions will support your mindful eating practice:

- ⊙ Be present—turn off all electronic devices while eating
- ⊙ Consciously focus on your food and imagine where it came from

Start by imagining the farm where it was planted, the rays of the sun, and the water that helped it flourish. Think about the farmer who grew it and the truck that shipped it to your store. Think about how the food was prepared, and how your body is absorbing it. This practice helps you slow down and be present. It can also give you a greater appreciation for food from local and organic sources.

- ⊙ Appreciate and notice the color, smell and texture of your food
- ⊙ Start each meal with three mindful breaths, and continue to focus on your breathing while you eat.
- ⊙ Stop at least two more times during your meal to take three more mindful breaths.

This will help refocus your attention to the present and give you an opportunity to reassess whether you're full or should continue eating. It sounds simple, and it is, yet it is an incredibly powerful technique to stay present and in control.

- ⊙ Check in with yourself before you eat more or get seconds

Before you head to the kitchen for another serving, actively ask yourself if you're really hungry and need more, or if you're simply eating out of habit.

Don't drink your calories

Most calories in drinks lack nutrients and are therefore "empty" calories. Sodas, most sport drinks and even 100% fruit juices are full of sugar, empty calories, and in some cases contain added, potentially harmful chemicals.

A single soda has 40 grams of sugar, more than double the sugar in ice cream! Half a cup of Häagen-Dazs vanilla ice cream has 14 grams of sugar, and even Ben and Jerry's Cherry Garcia has only 21 grams. A soda has 40 grams of sugar! There's just no reason for us to drink that.

Even something as simple as adding sugar to coffee or tea adds calories with no nutritional benefit and can send your blood glucose and insulin levels on a rollercoaster.

And when did a glorified chocolate milkshake become an acceptable coffee choice? That's good marketing, Starbucks! I can't argue with that success—at least, not as a shareholder. As a physician, I'm not impressed.

Remember, the purpose of drinking liquids is to nourish and hydrate your body. Water or herbal teas without sugar do this best and should be your mainstay.

TIP ◔ You don't have to quit sugar in your coffee cold turkey. Start by cutting the amount in half. Give your taste buds a couple of weeks to recalibrate, and you'll then be able to cut it in half again without noticing a big difference.

Unfortunately, diet sodas are not necessarily a healthy alternative.

Studies of aspartame in rats have persistently raised questions about increased cancer risk. Human studies have shown that aspartame increases insulin spikes equivalent to those caused by real sugar, and can even cause equivalent blood glucose spikes.

These results show how it is difficult to fool your brain. Your brain still registers the fake sweeteners as "sweet," which triggers the hormonal cascade leading to increased glucose and increased insulin, just as it would with real sugar.

That's probably why numerous studies have found links between diet soda intake and a higher risk of diabetes and obesity.

If you need an artificial sweetener, some marginal evidence suggests that stevia could be a better choice. There's no question, however, that you're better off simply skipping the sweetener altogether.

What about alcohol?

Some studies have suggested that mild to moderate alcohol intake may have mild health benefits. I would argue, however, that it still has minimal if any *nutritional* benefit, and can be high in simple sugars and calories. Therefore, drink alcohol only in small amounts for a healthy overall nutritional practice.

If you've done a great job avoiding added sugar during the day, you can even use a glass of wine or a scotch as your "reward." If you had one too many handfuls of the office candy jar, on the other hand, then you better stay away from alcohol that night.

What about juicing and smoothies?

The purpose of juicing and smoothies is to fill a nutritional need that you are not otherwise meeting with real foods. Don't assume they're healthy and that everyone should do it.

For example, if you can't get enough nutrients and calories from real foods, juices and smoothies can be a very good way to achieve better nutrition. Some people simply cannot stomach a salad full of spinach, kale, cauliflower, broccoli, avocado and so on. For them, throwing those ingredients in a juicer and adding something sweet like berries or an apple can be a good trick to get their veggies.

Smoothies with avocados, nut butters, or hemp seeds, can also be beneficial for those who need to add more protein and fat.

The danger from both juicing and smoothies is that it's too easy to load up on sugars, carbohydrates, and unnecessary calories. These drinks usually lack fiber, too, which is one of the most beneficial components of fruits and vegetables.

The bottom line: avoiding sugary, processed liquid calories like sodas and fruit juices is essential for reducing your sugar intake and improving your health. Use smoothies and juicing only when you can't get enough vegetables, fruit, protein or fat from real food during your day.

Recap of Best Practices

- ⊙ Eat real food
- ⊙ Eliminate added sugars
- ⊙ Make your meals vegetable-based
- ⊙ Eat natural monounsaturated fats
- ⊙ Avoid manufactured trans fats
- ⊙ Eat the minimum calories needed
- ⊙ Control your surroundings
- ⊙ Be mindful when you eat
- ⊙ Don't drink sugar

Areas of scientific controversy

Now let's get into the "meat" of the discussion. There is no shortage of disagreement in nutritional science. In this section, I'll share my assessment of the science and include lessons from my fifteen years of professional clinical experience.

Saturated fats and cholesterol

In previous decades, experts taught as fact that saturated fats and dietary cholesterol directly increased the risk of heart attack and stroke.

Now, that theory has fallen under intense scrutiny and, based on current evidence, is likely untrue. To understand this better, we need to understand the background of how the low-fat and low-cholesterol movement became popularized.

A Brief History of Fat & Cholesterol

Early health studies suggested that increased dietary cholesterol and saturated fat intake was associated with an increase in cardiovascular disease. This was most popularly noted with Dr. Ancel Keys' "Seven Countries Study" which started in the 1950s.

Dr. Keys believed that people in countries that ate foods high in cholesterol and saturated fat had higher rates of coronary heart disease, and those that ate less had lower rates. He concluded that dietary fat and cholesterol **caused** heart disease.

In 1968 the American Heart Association and Dr. Keys recommended that all individuals limit their dietary cholesterol and fat intake. The American government incorporated this recommendation into its official dietary guidelines in 1977.

Based on these guidelines, the medical profession defined a healthy diet as one that was low in fat and cholesterol. Food companies raced to the market with "healthy" low fat food, and a multi-million dollar food industry was born.

However, the problem was that Dr. Keys' study was purely observational. There was no control group, no randomization, and the study did not control for many essential variables other than fat and cholesterol consumption. Therefore, it could not prove causation. At best, it could merely point out an observed coincidence.

For instance, one of his main examples of low saturated fat intake correlating with low cardiac disease came from the Greek island of Crete.

Cretan subjects had a very low incidence of heart disease, and at the time he observed them, ate very little saturated fat. However, they were also manual laborers who performed strenuous physical labor for most of their lives. It's no surprise that they would have less heart disease than a more sedentary industrialized population. Perhaps their low incidence of heart disease had more to do with their lifelong physical activity, and nothing to do with their food intake. Keys' study did nothing to answer that question.

Dr. Keys' study also did not control for sugar intake, vegetable intake, stress management, social interactions and other factors that contribute to heart disease. For example, it's very plausible that people who ate more saturated fat also ate more burgers, more French fries, more simple carbohydrates (buns), more milk shakes, more soda, and fewer vegetables. As a result, it's very shortsighted to say with certainty that fat was the culprit.

Why did his study gain so much traction despite the faulty science?

President Dwight Eisenhower had just had a heart attack in 1955, and heart disease in the U.S. was becoming the nation's number one cause of death. Everyone was primed to find a scapegoat, and Dr. Keys was ready to give it to them.

From a psychological perspective, it makes sense that society wanted to find the silver bullet: the one thing they could do to avoid heart disease. Avoiding saturated fat and cholesterol seemed like that thing.

In addition, Big Business had a hand in the outcome. We now have evidence showing that the sugar industry systematically paid Harvard scientists to promote fat as the culprit, and to suppress science showing that sugar was a main contributor to heart disease. In essence, it was the perfect storm to promote dietary fat as the cause of all our ills.

This theory was also popularized by an underlying assumption that eating fat makes us become fat. After all, dietary fat and body fat are one and the same, right? Wrong!

But wait: if cholesterol and fat are found in plaques, the substances which clog arteries, then they must get there because we ate foods containing cholesterol and fat, right? Also wrong!

That thinking ignores the complex physiology involved in digesting food. It turns out that our bodies are more likely to convert sugar to fat, and less likely to store fat we eat. Sugar increases insulin levels, and insulin is a hormone that causes our bodies to store fat, and can lead to fatty plaques in our arteries. That's also likely why low-fat, higher-carbohydrate diets have consistently shown less weight loss than higher-fat, low-carbohydrate diets.

It seems contradictory, but eating fat can actually help us burn fat. As an example, a ketogenic diet, which is up to 80% fat and less than 20 grams of carbohydrate per day, is one of the best diets for fat loss. When insulin and glucose levels are low, our bodies preferentially burn fat even if we eat a high percentage of calories from fat.

It sounds implausible, but that's only because we have been incorrectly taught the opposite for decades. The science tells us that it is not only plausible—it is actual fact.

What about the studies that show that eating fat and cholesterol increase total cholesterol levels? Doesn't that mean that eating fat and cholesterol causes heart disease? No, it does not.

As it turns out, change in total cholesterol in response to diet is a poor marker for cardiovascular risk. The biggest danger likely occurs when LDL increases, inflammation increases, and HDL decreases. Most dietary saturated fat and cholesterol intake, on the other hand, increases HDL and LDL proportionately. The important HDL:LDL ratio therefore stays the same, thus likely *not* increasing the risk of cardiovascular disease.

More than fifty years have passed since the low-fat craze began. There are still no randomized controlled trials to support the hypothesis that dietary fat and cholesterol directly increase the risk for heart disease. In fact, multiple health studies have shown no correlation between dietary cholesterol intake and cardiovascular risk.

To be fair, plenty of observational studies and meta analyses continue to suggest a relationship. But again, they cannot prove causation. Most of these studies cannot adequately control for the fact that traditional saturated fat eaters will also eat more fried foods, more simple carbohydrates, more sugars, more processed food, and fewer vegetables than control subjects.

Compellingly, the American College of Cardiology (ACC) finally reversed their ban on dietary cholesterol in 2014, saying that "There is insufficient evidence to determine whether lowering dietary cholesterol reduces LDL-C."

In 2015, U.S. federal guidelines followed suit, saying that "Available evidence shows no appreciable relationship between consumption of dietary cholesterol and serum cholesterol."

••

My Ideal Research Study

I've actually designed the study I wish researchers would conduct to answer this question. Check the Book Resources Blog at DrBretScher.com to practice your scientific study design mastery, and let me know what you think!

••

In conclusion, no high-level evidence proves that we should avoid animal-based foods. The science is split on whether or not there is even an association, and there is certainly no causative proof.

Does that mean you should have a porterhouse steak wrapped in bacon with every meal? Of course not. There are no good studies showing that saturated fat directly *reduces* heart attacks, either. Meanwhile, animal fats and proteins can definitely be an enjoyable addition to an otherwise plant-based way of eating.

If you choose not to eat animal products for ethical or environmental reasons, that admirable personal choice may benefit your health and the health of the earth.

As we've discussed, there is no doubt that real, fresh vegetables (from the earth!) in a variety of colors should make up the majority of every meal.

If you enjoy a vegan diet and can get adequate protein, omega-3 fats, B vitamins, iron, and calcium while limiting your sugars and simple grains, and don't find meal planning and preparation burdensome, by all means go for it! Eating animal products is unlikely to offer you many additional health benefits.

The problem is that only a comparatively few people can manage to eat this way.

Animal food sources are the most efficient way to get required amounts of protein, B12, calcium, iron, omega-3 fatty acids, and other important nutrients.

Allowing fish, meat, chicken and eggs in your meals simplifies your food planning and preparation. For many, it helps create a fun, enjoyable and satisfying eating pattern that is sustainable for the long term.

So don't stress about avoiding animal food sources.

As I'll explain below, focus instead on appropriate proportions of high quality animal fats and proteins as part of a real food, plant-based way of eating.

If you make it a priority, you'll be able to find responsibly raised animal food sources that benefit your health and the health of the earth. Plus, you'll assure yourself of the best food nature has to offer.

The Danger in Not Eating Fat

If we traditionally weren't supposed to eat fat, what were we supposed to eat instead?

Unfortunately, the recommendation to adopt a low-fat and low-cholesterol diet spawned an entire industry of high-carbohydrate and high-sugar foods ranging from cookies and cakes to meat alternatives. Supposedly "healthy" hydrogenated (solid) vegetable oils were recommended to replace anything that had dietary fat and cholesterol.

As a result, high-sugar, high-fructose, processed foods became the new staple of the American diet.

Sugary cereals, bagels and muffins replaced eggs for breakfast. Orange juice and other sugary drinks replaced whole milk. White bread and white flour noodles replaced meat and chicken.

Since that time, obesity and diabetes have increased dramatically. In 1950, 12% of Americans were obese. In 1980, it increased slightly to 15%, and then skyrocketed to 35% by 2000. At the same time, rates of heart disease and other chronic illnesses have continued to climb.

This doesn't prove that the flood of low-fat high-carb foods were the cause, but it certainly shows that the low-fat shift did not achieve the intended result of improving our health.

At best, the recommendation to avoid fat failed to make us healthy. At worst, it directly caused an explosion of obesity, diabetes, autoimmune disease, and other chronic illness.

It turns out, adding fat to our meals helps us feel full, reduces our carbohydrate cravings, and actually leads us to eat fewer calories during the day. Fat, therefore, should be a healthy addition to our meals, and not something to be avoided.

We can only wonder how different our lives might be today if the sugar hypothesis of heart disease, rather than the fat hypothesis, had been adopted in the 1960s.

• •

Fat: The Word We Whisper

The theory of fat as universally bad has infiltrated our language more than we realize. In fact, "fat" has become one of the most charged words in our language.

Think about it. "Sugar" is a term of affection. You can hear the waitress with her southern drawl saying, "Hey, sugar. What can I get you?" We frequently use "sweet" to mean nice, caring, kind. "She's so sweet."

"Fat," on the other hand, is a word you have to whisper for fear someone will hear you. It's become associated with things that are ugly, unpleasant, and unhealthy.

It's time to reverse that association and realize that dietary fat is a vital component of healthy nutrition.

• •

Gluten

If you read popular media reports and celebrity endorsements, you'll likely conclude that everyone should be gluten-free. After all, if New England Patriots quarterback Tom Brady is doing it, shouldn't I? Before you swear off gluten for good, however, let's look at the data.

Gluten is a protein found in wheat, barley and rye, and in foods made with those grains, like bread and pasta.

In people with the medical condition of celiac disease, or gluten-sensitive enteropathy, the body sees gluten as a foreign invader and is unable to properly absorb it. In addition, gluten stimulates the body to mount an autoimmune response against the lining of the intestines. This causes significant intestinal damage and malabsorption of necessary nutrients.

Symptoms of celiac disease include abdominal pain, bloating, and rashes. It can also cause anemia, bone problems, and malnutrition. Your doctor can diagnose celiac disease with a blood test and a biopsy of your small intestine.

Without question, those with proven celiac disease must avoid gluten. Fortunately, that is the least common gluten-related issue people deal with.

More commonly, people are sensitive to gluten even though they don't have celiac disease. They simply find that they feel much better when they avoid gluten-containing foods. They have more energy, less bloating, clearer skin, and some even think and concentrate better. If you're in this camp, there's likewise little controversy that you should avoid gluten. After all, our bodies do not require gluten for good health.

I'll emphasize again: our bodies need proteins and fats, vitamins and minerals. There is no physiological need for gluten. If it makes you feel poorly, there is no need to eat it.

What if you tolerate gluten without negative effects? Should you still avoid or limit it?

The literature does not support being overly strict about eliminating gluten for all individuals. After all, the Mediterranean diet, which has been shown to reduce the risk of cardiovascular disease, relies on reasonable portions of pasta and whole grains. The key here is "reasonable" portion sizes. The average portion of pasta in Europe is about half a cup. Most U.S. restaurants serve four times that much!

However, when we look back at the overall goals of nutrition, we find that mass-produced bread, pasta, baked goods and other gluten-containing items usually satisfy very few of those goals.

They can be enjoyable, but that's often their only benefit. These products tend to be more processed and contain more sugar. They provide few if any necessary nutrients. They aren't as filling and they frequently lack healthy fats.

For these reasons alone, it makes sense to minimize gluten-containing foods in a healthy nutritional lifestyle.

I usually recommend that you simply try limiting or outright eliminating gluten for two weeks. During that period, get your carbohydrates mainly from vegetables and fruits, with a smaller amount of whole or complex grains such as quinoa or millet.

After your two-week trial, decide if you felt better. Did you lose weight more easily? Did you have more energy? Or did you miss the gluten-containing foods so much that it out outweighed the benefits? It's then up to you to decide whether or not to make it part of your healthy nutritional practice.

TIP ◗ Even though gluten itself does not have any beneficial nutrients, the food containing gluten may. These foods are frequently fiber-rich and fortified with B vitamins, iron and other nutrients. If you eliminate gluten, make sure you're getting proper nutrients from the foods you do eat. If you are choosing mostly Mediterranean-style, vegetable-based real foods with appropriate proportions of high quality animal fats and proteins, then you'll have no problem.

Finally, answer me this: Why does every restaurant serve bread to start your meal? Why would we want to fill up on a simple carbohydrate with few if any nutritional benefits before we get the meal that we actually chose and are paying for? It doesn't make nutritional sense. Skip the bread, and enjoy the real food—the nutrient-dense foods, the vegetables, healthy fats and proteins. Your enjoyment *and* your health will thank you!

Vegetarianism

Here is a very common conversation I have with my patients and clients.

Me: "Tell me about your nutrition."

Client: "Don't worry, doc. I'm as healthy as they come. I'm a vegetarian."

Should I stop there and take him at his word that since he's a vegetarian he's "as healthy as they come?" Of course not!

It may sound counterintuitive, but being a vegetarian does not necessarily mean making healthy, plant-based food choices. After all, a huge plate of spaghetti with processed and heavily refined tomato sauce is perfectly vegetarian. A tofu burger on a huge bun with ketchup is perfectly vegetarian. Yet those meals are a far cry from a healthy, vegetable-based nutritional pattern.

Studies on vegetarians have shown a higher likelihood of vitamin and protein deficiencies, as well as higher consumption of grains and simple carbohydrates.

In fact, no *randomized* trials show that vegetarian diets reduce the risk of heart attacks or death. People frequently cite Dr. Dean Ornish's work to support the claim that a vegetarian diet can reverse heart disease. However, he has never published a dietary intervention trial that shows the effects specifically of a vegetarian diet.

Dr. Ornish *has* shown that when people quit smoking, improve their exercise, practice stress management, and follow a vegetarian nutritional pattern, they can halt or reverse the progression of coronary artery disease.

That is a powerful finding, and I do not want to minimize the importance of his work. However, it is important to emphasize that there were many interventions, not just vegetarian food choices. So we cannot claim the vegetarian diet was any more or less important than quitting smoking, exercising, or practicing stress management.

To be fair, observational studies also show that on average, vegetarians are healthier than meat eaters. Once again, we can't prove cause and effect as they also tend to make other healthy choices. But they're probably consuming more vegetables, and that's always a good idea.

A vegetarian diet that's vegetable-based, low in sugar and simple carbohydrates, with adequate fat, protein and vitamins is likely an ideal diet for those can maintain this way of eating long-term.

But even vegetarians need to remember the most important rule of nutrition: just eat real food!

Calorie restriction

There's an old saying that "Calorie restriction may or may not make you live longer, but it certainly makes your life feel longer!"

Restricting your caloric intake to 1,500 calories per day is not an easy or very enjoyable task for most people, and the likelihood of maintaining that pattern over many years is very low. But is there a compelling reason to even consider it?

It turns out, there just might be. Numerous studies have shown that restricting caloric intake while ensuring adequate nutrition significantly increases the lifespan of many different species, from cellular organisms all the way up to primates like monkeys and apes.

The application to humans has not been definitively proven, but the science is very encouraging. While it's not entirely clear how calorie restriction extends longevity, it may be that it results in better glucose utilization and insulin sensitivity, and reduces cellular oxidation. The beneficial effects have even been seen on a genetic level.

In fact, caloric restriction seems to be the closest thing to the fountain of youth that anyone has found to date. For most, though, it just isn't practical as we strive to maintain our quality of life.

That's where intermittent fasting (IF) comes in. Intermittent fasting helps you get most of the benefits of calorie restriction without dramatically altering your lifestyle or making yourself miserable.

Intermittent fasting is not a conventional diet where you only eat certain foods. It's a pattern of eating. It doesn't change *what* you eat, it changes when you eat. You still need to eat healthy, nutrient-dense food when you do eat. This is important from an overall health perspective, but also so that you stay full and can fast with greater ease.

Intermittent fasting can also lead to easier weight loss. Dr. Jason Fung's excellent book *The Complete Guide to Fasting* goes into the science in detail. My focus, however, is on the overall health benefits above and beyond weight loss. Remember, when we make healthy lifestyle choices, appropriate weight loss will naturally follow.

....

Mini-Meals: Pros & Cons

Many people hear "fasting" and shriek "Fasting?! Are you crazy?! I need to eat every 3-4 hours to keep from getting hungry and to regulate my blood sugar! I would be miserable if I fasted." For some people, this statement may be true. For many, it's not actually the case.

The theory of frequent small meals has been popularized so much—even with a lack of scientific evidence—that many people feel it is absolute truth. But the truth is that there is no one strategy that works for all of us.

If you get shaky and hungry if you don't eat frequently, mini-meals every two hours might work well. Just remember to plan ahead so you're constantly surrounded by good healthy food choices. Otherwise, you're likely to grab whatever's around, which tends to be higher-carbohydrate, more processed foods.

If your workplace is like mine, you'll have to plan for an extra level of preparation to make sure you have better choices available for your mini-meals. After all, what do they have available in the doctor's lounges of most hospitals? Muffins, bagels, chips, and cereals. I'm not sure if that's ironic or just sad.

If you instead focus on more complex carbohydrates and more fats, you'll find that you stay full longer. You won't have the rapid blood sugar and insulin swings, and won't feel the need to eat as frequently.

The mini-meal strategy can also lead to "calorie creep," where your mini-meals start to get bigger and bigger and the calories add up.

• •

Intermittent fasting is based on good scientific evidence demonstrating that it helps promote fat loss while maintaining lean body mass, and even has beneficial effects on markers for diabetes. It also requires less planning, less shopping and less worry than eating frequent small meals.

Here's a brief overview of how intermittent fasting works. When our bodies go without food for a certain period of time, we start breaking down our own body fat into ketones. Ketones are natural substances we can use instead of sugar for energy. In fact, we can make energy more efficiently from ketones than from sugar.

However, we only reach this fasting state on average 12 hours after our last meal. So if you stop eating at 8 p.m. and eat breakfast the following morning at 6 a.m., only ten hours have passed. Your body never reached the fasting state and therefore never started to burn fat.

Intermittent fasting requires establishing an eating "window" and a fasting "window." The most common and easiest approach is simply to delay eating for several hours after you wake up. Just make lunch your first meal of the day.

Say you decide that your eating window is noon to 7 p.m. During that time you have lunch, possibly a snack, and dinner. Your fasting window, during which you eat nothing, will then begin at 7 p.m. and end at noon the next day.

On this schedule, your body will be in a true fasting state 12 hours after you last ate, around 7 a.m. During this period, your body will start to preferentially burn fat as a fuel source, thereby increasing fat loss and suppressing your glucose and insulin levels.

Keep in mind that you still need to get adequate calories and nutrients during the day. If you can't control when you'll be able to eat or what will be available to eat, you may have trouble getting enough high-quality calories. That's why it's important to practice intermittent fasting on days when you have more control over your schedule and your food. On days where your schedule's not your own, eat breakfast as usual to avoid stress about finding a high-quality lunch at the right time.

This schedule offers another benefit. Eliminating eating after 7 p.m. also eliminates many of the poor food decisions we make. Think about your late-night snacks. Are they veggie-based, nutrient-dense foods? Or are they more likely carbohydrate-rich, sweetened, low-nutrient foods?

It's okay, you don't have to answer that one out loud. I've seen what people (including me!) eat after 7 p.m. It's not pretty.

The Goldilocks Principle

Intermittent fasting helps you calibrate the amount you eat on "normal" days so that you eat just the right amount needed to feel great—not too much, not too little. Experimenting with a nutrient tracking app like My Fitness Pal is a great way to educate yourself about how much you need to eat to feel great. This helps you keep track of your calories and percentages of protein, fat and carbohydrates. Don't worry about hitting targets or certain percentages when you start using this. Use the tool simply to compare your IF days to your "normal" days. You can also compare your "slip days" to your "good days."

4: NOURISH YOUR BODY

For instance, if your carbohydrate percentages are higher on your IF days, you might realize that you need to control your environment better on those days by making healthy fats and proteins more readily available.

Or you may find that your calories are a third less on your IF days, yet your energy and sense of satisfaction are just as good as your non-fasting days. That suggests you're eating more than you need to on non-fasting days.

I don't recommend that you count your calories all the time. That is far too stressful and too much work. I do suggest you get a feel for how much food is the right amount for you. Try this exercise for a couple of weeks. It'll be incredibly educational and will help you adjust your portion sizes throughout the day.

....

I've found that almost everyone can successfully implement and maintain intermittent fasting. It requires very little behavior change, and it's powerful enough that it will actually make a difference. You simply have to change the timing of your meals.

In addition, you may find that you enjoy not worrying about what's for breakfast, especially if you're busy in the morning getting the kids ready for school or getting yourself to work.

Intermittent fasting provides another, unexpected, payoff: the psychological benefit of realizing that "I am in control of food and hunger. Hunger is not in control of me." This is a crucial change in our mindset. Knowing we're in control of, rather than being controlled by, our hunger is invaluable for implementing healthy lifestyle practices.

Your brain and your body adapt to your state of hunger. You learn that you don't need to immediately react to hunger by snacking on whatever's available. You don't have to overeat to make up for the hunger. You can remain mindful and in control of your actions.

A common saying is that "diets are easy in the contemplation, difficult in the execution. Intermittent fasting is difficult in the contemplation but easy in the execution."

Put another way, it's easy to decide to go on a traditional diet, but hard to maintain it. Intermittent fasting is just the opposite: it's hard to decide to try it, but surprisingly easy to do it and maintain it.

The more experience you have with fasting, the easier it becomes, and the more you realize it's just fine to be a little hungry. You gain control of your hunger, and your body reaps the benefits of lower glucose and insulin levels. That's a powerful combination for reducing the risk of chronic diseases.

Sodium & salt

You've probably heard the advice that we all need to limit sodium intake for healthy nutrition. I know I've heard it and unfortunately said it many times during my early career.

The latest science, however, suggests that most people don't need to restrict salt use. In fact, extremely *high* sodium intake is potentially beneficial for high-performance athletes at risk for excessive sweating, and it would be dangerous for them to limit sodium intake.

Those with poorly controlled hypertension, a weakened heart muscle, or congestive heart failure do need to control their sodium intake. If this describes you, talk to your physician before increasing your salt intake.

People who are sensitive to sodium should also follow a low-sodium diet. These individuals tend to retain fluid or experience dramatic increases in blood pressure when their diet contains sodium. To see if you're sodium-sensitive, check your blood pressure and watch for swelling in your ankles.

If you are not in the above-mentioned categories, then sodium restriction provides no benefit for you, and may actually be harmful.

It turns out that current nutritional guidelines and the American Heart Association's recommendation that adults limit sodium intake to 2300 milligrams/ day (about a teaspoon of table salt) originated from a single 30-day trial, the DASH trial. This was a trial of only 460 individuals, first reported in 1997.

The DASH trial found that lowering salt below 2300 milligrams reduced blood pressure—but by only 5 points, hardly an earth-shattering result.

Moreover, the trial was so short that no data could be gathered on the effect of sodium reduction on clinical outcomes like heart attacks or strokes. Once again, a government guideline that shaped medical dogma came from very limited data.

Two separate meta-analysis studies concluded that salt intake was linked to a U-shaped outcome. This means that there was an increase in cardiovascular events at both extremely high *and* low levels of sodium intake.

Moreover, in 2013, an Institute of Medicine committee stated officially that there was no scientific reason to recommend less than 2300mg of daily sodium intake.

And not a single study conducted in the last fifteen years has shown a link between reduced sodium consumption and reduction of heart attacks, strokes, or death.

Studies have indeed suggested that lower salt intake may slightly reduce blood pressure, but that reduction didn't translate to better clinical outcomes like fewer heart attacks.

Instead, it's similar to the pattern I described earlier for saturated fat consumption: it indeed may raise total cholesterol in some people, but that doesn't translate into more heart attacks, strokes or deaths.

You should, however, consider the quality of your salt. Refined table salt can be thought of in the same way as refined, processed sugar. It has been stripped of its nutrients and minerals, and provides little if any nutritional or health benefit.

Celtic sea salt, Himalayan salt, and a product aptly named Real Salt, on the other hand, are minimally processed. They're full of minerals and nutrients that our bodies need. Yes, salt can actually have a positive impact on our health!

The best way to eat

Is there a best way to eat? The research suggests that the answer is yes, the Mediterranean pattern of eating based on real foods.

This way of eating emphasizes fish, avocados, nuts, olive oil, vegetables and fruit. It allows poultry and low-fat plain dairy, consumes red meat sparingly, and avoids sweets, baked goods, and processed foods. It focuses on quality ingredients and controlled portions, especially for grains and simple carbohydrates. Importantly, it honors the principle of eating to nourish your body.

With this approach, there's no reason to avoid high-quality fats or high-quality salt. These elements add enjoyment without any proven risks.

Initial interest in the Mediterranean diet began when researchers noted that people living along the Mediterranean Sea in Greece, Spain and Italy had less cardiovascular disease even though their diets were higher in fat.

Subsequent investigations published as the now-famous Lyon Heart Study and the PREDIMED study demonstrated that a Mediterranean-style diet reduced the risk of early death, cardiovascular diseases, diabetes, and lowered the oxidation of plaque-causing cholesterol. In fact, the Lyon study reported significant reductions in heart attacks, cardiac deaths, and overall deaths after less than four years of follow-up.

Yes, you read that correctly. A single dietary intervention reduced the risk of death in less than four years!

That's an impressive resume for a single intervention. If a new drug showed those results, we'd see a multi-million dollar marketing campaign promoting its use to physicians and consumers alike.

But this isn't a drug. Instead, it's just a pattern of eating. Nobody owns it, and therefore companies cannot patent it and profit from it. That's why it's up to each of us to choose this lifestyle as our medicine, and as a better path to natural health free of drugs.

Notice that none of this research focused on a single nutrient or a single food type.

Instead, it investigated a cultural style of eating, with many different dimensions. It went beyond just the types of foods they ate or did not eat. It included appropriate portion sizes, the freshness and quality of ingredients, and the social environment and mindset of the individuals as they ate.

That point is worth reiterating. The Mediterranean diet pattern that reduced cardiovascular death and heart attacks included high-quality real foods, and it also included the culture of eating, appropriate portion sizes, and presumably a more relaxed and more mindful approach to eating.

Can we say which of these elements was most important? Is it perhaps the combination that's most powerful?

In the end, it may not matter: integration of the Mediterranean diet research with the scientific consensus on nutrition detailed earlier creates a powerful intersection of knowledge to help guide our nutritional choices.

As I said before, we don't eat proteins, fats and carbohydrates. We eat food, itself a complicated combination of "healthy" and "unhealthy" ingredients.

Saying we should eat more fat without further context is not helpful. But incorporating that advice into a Mediterranean style of eating gives us a practical roadmap for an effective nutritional strategy.

NEXT STEPS

Modify your mindset

Food is meant to nourish our body, provide energy, and keep us from getting hungry. Once we have met those requirements, we need to stop eating.

This is unfortunately a serious issue in American society. We have truly become a "supersize" culture.

Our standard portion sizes are enormous compared to most other countries. Our concept of "normal" has been so distorted that the concept of moderation has little meaning to most Americans.

We have to reverse this mindset and eat for nourishment. We then have to stop when we've met that goal. It doesn't mean we can't enjoy our meals, or eat socially. But it does mean we have to remain mindful of our portion sizes and their dramatic impact on our health.

Studies show that hunter-gatherer tribes consistently avoid the chronic diseases that plague industrialized societies. Why? Quite possibly because the relative scarcity of food prevents them from over-eating. Eating until they can eat no more has never become part of their culture.

They follow the practice of eating for nourishment and fulfillment. They eat until they have met those goals and then they stop. That style of eating alone would greatly reduce obesity and blood sugar related chronic illnesses.

We can only maintain healthy eating patterns if we are purposeful and mindful about our nutrition. That means rethinking all of our assumptions, our traditions and our practices around eating. It may sound daunting—but most of us have never thought about it before. Once we set our minds to it, we quickly find it's achievable.

The first step is recognizing the need. Do you need to eat bread before your meal is served? Do you need to dip your hand in the office candy bowl as you walk by? Do you need that second helping while you're socializing around the dinner table? Do you need the sugary coffee with whipped cream, or would a simple coffee do the trick? As you go through your day, find the areas where you can question your norms and your patterns to help reframe your mindset towards health.

Eat 100% real food

Your nutrition plan calls for two one-week trials of eating 100% real food. That means everything you eat for those weeks should be **REAL** food. Nothing processed, nothing with added sugars, nothing from a bag or box, unless it's a bag or box of fresh veggies.

Vegetables & fruit

When eating 100% real food, most of what you eat comes from vegetables and fruits.

Remember, choose mostly non-starchy vegetables like these:

- Spinach
- Kale
- Chard
- Broccoli
- Cauliflower
- Zucchini
- Mushrooms
- Onions
- Asparagus
- Tomatoes

Choose some, but fewer, starchy veggies like these:

- Sweet potato
- Butternut squash
- Beets
- Corn
- Peas

All fruit is fair game, especially lower-glycemic fruits like berries, apples, pears, plums, oranges, and grapefruit. Eat fewer servings of dried fruit and higher-glycemic fruit, like raisins, pineapple, watermelon, and dates.

Healthy fats

Make a concerted effort to add natural healthy fats like avocados, mixed nuts and olives to your meals and snacks. True, olive oil is processed—but it's still a single ingredient, so it still counts as 100% real food. Think of it as the perfect salad dressing, and the perfect sauce for chicken and meat. No hidden sugar, fillers or additives!

Nut butters are another great choice—just make sure their only ingredients are nuts and salt. Check labels carefully for added sugar.

Animal protein

The other main component of real-food nutrition is animal protein. Keep your meals veggie-based, but feel free to add eggs, chicken, beef, pork, milk and cheese. Prepare them simply. Avoid sauces with added sugar and fillers.

And that's it. 100% real food.

What's missing?

You'll notice quite a few things missing from these recommendations. There's nothing processed. No grains, no bread, no pasta, no rice, no crackers, no cookies, no muffins, no cereal.

Everything is its own ingredient.

If you're already starting to dread a lifetime without bread, remember: you don't have to do this forever. I'm asking that you do this only twice, for just one week at a time, during Week #2 and Week #4.

My goal is for you to experience how differently you can feel following real food nutrition. It may be challenging at first, but it's just a week—you can do it! And the second week will likely be even easier.

You'll feel better, be healthier—and you'll be much more aware of how many processed foods you've been eating.

When your two weeks are over and you go back to your standard way of eating, you may realize that you don't need the bread before dinner. You don't need the big plate of pasta when you can have a big plate of veggies and a small side of pasta. And you'll realize that berries, apples and a little nut butter make for a fantastic dessert.

Stay focused, remember your goals, banish any negative thoughts, and go for it. You can do this!

Forget old-school "diets"

If getting to a healthy weight is a concern for you, you've likely considered various "diets." I would argue that we can do much better on our own through more comprehensive lifestyle changes than we can with traditional weight loss programs.

A study of commercial weight loss programs in 2015 found that only Weight Watchers and Jenny Craig had any significant success at helping participants maintain weight loss for more than one year. Even then, participants were only able to achieve a 5% weight loss at the one-year mark.

Lifestyle changes produce gradual, lasting results that are easier to sustain in the long term. A 10-pound weight loss in a week is worthless if you gain it all back a month later.

What matters for your health is that you establish healthy patterns of living and eating that you can maintain over the course of your life.

Life is a marathon, not a sprint.

Food quality matters

We also need to focus on the fact that food quality matters. One of the problems in the standard American diet may be that the quality of our animal-based foods has deteriorated as a result of mass production and the associated use of corn feeds, antibiotics and hormones.

Studies have clearly shown higher nutrient content and lower toxin content in grass-fed rather than grain-fed meat, wild as opposed to farmed fish, pasture-raised instead of pen-raised chicken and hens.

From an evolutionary perspective, our ancestors only ate grass-fed meat. They only caught wild fish. They only ate eggs from hens freely grazing. Our bodies have evolved over thousands of years to eat this way. If we could get back to those basics, we would take a huge step towards restoring a healthier dietary pattern.

Imagine you have two meals in front of you, equal in size and content. One has fewer toxins, more nutrients, and is better for the earth. Which one would you choose?

We can do our part to help ourselves and protect Mother Earth by purposely patronizing companies and restaurants that provide responsibly raised, grass-fed cattle, organic antibiotic-free chicken, and eggs from pasture-raised hens. Some of my favorites here in San Diego include Whole Foods, True Food Kitchen, Tender Greens and Flower Child. The cost may be more, but it is a small price to pay to help protect our health and our planet.

CONCLUSION

Nourishing our bodies requires us to rethink all our assumptions and our individual and cultural traditions regarding food intake. Nourish your body with purpose, and your intention will translate into every aspect of your life.

Remember that everything we consume either benefits our health or hurts our health. Which one applies to what you're about to eat?

We need to choose our food for the purpose it is intended: to nourish, to relieve hunger, and to provide energy. We need to eat to eliminate hunger, not to feel stuffed.

By being mindful as we eat, by being present with our meal, we can control the urge to overeat, appreciate our food, and understand the benefits that food provides.

Controlling our surroundings means that we don't have to rely exclusively on self-control throughout the entire day.

In my experience, when you follow healthy nutritional practices, appropriate weight loss will follow. Plan ahead to increase your chances for success.

You'll make great strides in improving your nutrition for your health as you embrace these mindful tenets and the nutritional practices outlined above.

Not for a week, not for a month, but for your lifetime.

THE PLAN: NOURISH YOUR BODY

Week 1

⊙   Become more mindful with everything you eat. Ask yourself, what nutrition does it provide? Does it help you feel full and feel energized? Do you enjoy it? Does it help you or hurt you?

⊙ Practice mindful techniques when you eat. Start each meal with three mindful breaths, and focus on your food as you eat. Use this to help you assess your fullness, so you stop eating when you're no longer hungry.

Week 2

⊙ Make this a week of eating 100% real food. You need to see how good you can feel with a 100% real food diet.

⊙ Everything you eat should be from the earth or an animal, not a factory. Focus on real food, real veggies and real proteins/fats.

⊙ Detox your kitchen. Focus on the quality of what surrounds you. Control your environment by eliminating all non-real food, sweets, liquid calories, added sugars, and processed food.

⊙ It's just for a week. You can do it!

Week 3

⊙ Experiment with intermittent fasting one or two days per week. The easiest way is to stop eating at 6 or 7 p.m. Don't eat again until noon the next day.

⊙ Learn that you can control your hunger physically and psychologically.

⊙ Use a nutrient tracker like My Fitness Pal to track calories, protein, fat and carbohydrates. Don't worry about hitting targets or certain percentages. This is for your information only.

Week 4

⊙ Research potential restaurants where you can comfortably eat out.

⊙ Pick two or three "go to" restaurants and one or two menu items that work for your real food eating plan.

⊙ Repeat your week of 100% real food and see how much easier it is a second time.

For journal citations and more insight into the numerous nutritional studies and other research discussed in this chapter, visit the Book Resources Blog at DrBretScher.com.

5: Move With A Purpose

Here's the secret to moving with a purpose....move more!

Studies on longevity consistently point to one thing about activity: those who lived the longest moved their bodies the most during the day. They weren't necessarily competitive runners, and they didn't spend 30 minutes a day on the treadmill. They remained active for most of the day and simply moved their bodies. That's a goal we should all hope to achieve.

Of course, science tells us that planned, purposeful exercise is also very beneficial. For the greatest benefit, we need to combine exercise with an intentionally active lifestyle.

We shouldn't really need science to tell us that, and apparently the earliest physician, Hippocrates, didn't either, since he said around 400 BC that "Walking is man's best medicine."

However, sometimes it seems that society is conspiring against us. Our technology-driven world has created millions of sedentary jobs where we sit for hours in front of a computer screen. Then, in our free time, we spend yet more time with our computers, tablets, phones, video games, and televisions, again keeping us in one place without moving.

Add longer commutes and busy lives, and it's no wonder that most of us feel like we don't have enough time for exercise or physical activity.

Our "advanced" society has become a leading cause of the obesity and diabetes epidemic and of many chronic illnesses. It even led to the new slogan, "Sitting is the new smoking."

Fortunately, inactivity is one of the easiest issues to correct, once you know what to do.

THE EVIDENCE FOR EXERCISE

No scientific studies existed when Hippocrates proclaimed "Walking is man's best medicine." Today, we do have the science to back up this claim. We also have answers to other important questions, like "How much should I exercise?"

Exercise cuts early deaths & heart risk

Unlike prescription medications, which come with specific dosing instructions, exercise as a prescription can seem more nebulous. After all, there's no label telling us how much or how often. The Centers for Disease Control recommends:

- ⊙ At least 150 minutes of moderate activity per week OR
- ⊙ 75 minutes per week of high-intensity activity

These are reasonable goals, but they are not the only worthwhile goals.

I have many clients who say, "I can't find the time to do the whole 150 minutes per week, so why bother? I'm just setting myself up for failure."

Fortunately, research shows that it doesn't take much physical activity to reduce your risk of early death.

A 2015 study of about 600,000 middle-aged adults found that the highest risk of death was in those who did not exercise at all.

Even a "little amount" of exercise—more than zero, but less than 150 minutes each week—reduced the risk of death by 20%. The more study participants exercised, the more they reduced their risk of early death, up to a plateau of 450 minutes each week.

Exercise Effects on Risk of Early Death

Amount of Weekly Exercise	Cardiovascular & Mortality Result
No exercise or sedentary	Highest death rate and cardiovascular risk
Less than 150 minutes	Reduced deaths by 20% over sedentary
150 minutes	Reduced deaths by 31%
450 minutes	Reduced deaths by 39%
More than 450 min	No additional benefit, but no increased harm either

Another study, the Copenhagen Heart Study, also found that "light" exercise—running, in this case—even just once per week lowered the risk of early death. Clearly, even if you can't reach the 150-minute goal, just getting out there and being active still provides significant benefits.

Do you want to know the best part? Physical activity reduces your risk of death and, unlike medications, the only side effects are more energy, feeling stronger, improved thinking, and a better mood.

Does 5 minutes of running save lives?

The catchy headlines about a 2014 study declared that "As Little As 5 Minutes of Daily Running Saves Lives." Was it true?

This study followed over 55,000 men in their 40s, mostly white, for 15 years.

The study compared people who ran some, but less than 51 minutes each week, to non-runners. Overall, any amount of running, even as little as five minutes, was associated with a 30% lower death rate.

So does five minutes of running save lives? That conclusion is a bit of a stretch, since observational studies cannot completely correct for every possible factor that could affect outcomes.

But this study does suggest that we still benefit from a minimal amount of daily activity. I can't stress the importance of that enough! Just make your first goal being active, and you've already taken the first step at reducing your risk of death.

How about 1 minute of intense exercise?

Another study followed 25 sedentary people for six weeks. Researchers randomly assigned participants to either a control group that did no activity, a sprint interval training group (SIT), or a medium-intensity cardio training group (MICT).

The SIT group exercised for a total of nine minutes, with only one minute of maximum intensity broken up as three sets of 20 seconds each.

The MICT group cycled for 45 minutes at moderate intensity, defined as 70% of their maximum predicted heart rate.

What happened? The SIT and MICT groups both decreased their body fat and improved their oxygen uptake by almost 20%, an important fitness indicator. Surprisingly, the SIT participants also improved their insulin sensitivity, while the MICT group did not.

This was a powerful indicator that increasing the intensity of exercise has significant benefits, even for short exercise bouts. Since lack of time is the number one excuse for a lack of regular physical activity, this study is a welcome addition.

The bottom line

The take-home message from all these studies is that *any* amount of exercise reduces the risk of early death compared to inactivity.

No more excuses! Get out there and be active for as little or as much time as you have.

Even if you can't get the recommended 150 minutes per week, you can still improve your health and reduce your risk of obesity, diabetes, heart disease, and early death simply by moving your body regularly and getting some amount of exercise.

It doesn't get much more powerful than that!

NEXT STEPS

Modify your mindset

If you're not currently active, establishing an exercise routine can seem intimidating, time consuming, and very difficult.

The first step is to work on your mindset. Your goal is to get to the point where you believe that exercising and being active is "part of who I am."

Start with visualizing your goal. Then visualize the habits that you'll do to maintain your goal. Once you see where you want to go, getting there becomes that much easier.

- ⊙ How do you become more active during your day?
- ⊙ What does your exercise routine look like?
- ⊙ What makes it fun?
- ⊙ What makes it social?
- ⊙ When do you exercise?
- ⊙ Who do you exercise with?
- ⊙ How does it feel to exercise?
- ⊙ What do you expect to achieve?

To reach that goal, move with purpose. A low-intensity 20-minute elliptical workout will often leave you frustrated, wondering why you're not getting the results you want.

If you've had this experience, you might benefit from working with a personal trainer or in a group exercise class. Choose a trainer whose goal is to teach you the right exercises for your goals so you can do them independently, not someone who wants to keep you coming back week after week.

Last, know that your actions have a greater purpose. Setting an alarm to get up and walk every 60 minutes at work may seem like an inconvenient burden. Yet when you reframe your thought process and acknowledge that the small act of simply standing up and walking for a few minutes actually reduces your risk of dying, it suddenly becomes less of an inconvenience. Instead, you'll wonder why you haven't been doing this your entire life!

Park like you own a Tesla

What do we call the parking spaces right up front, nearest the entrance?

"Rock Star Parking."

We celebrate the ability to find the closest parking space. This is the opposite of what we should do!

One of my clients told me that the best thing he did for his heath was buying a Tesla. He explained that Teslas are very nice, very expensive cars, and you want to make sure no one's going to ding your car in tight parking spots.

They're also bigger than the average car, so my client had to start parking farther away to find an appropriate "Tesla parking space." He noticed that his daily steps on his FitBit started increasing without any conscious effort. And he started enjoying the extra one or two minutes from his car to the office, or from his car to the restaurant. They gave him a chance to breathe and think while he moved his body.

Thank you, Elon Musk!

We can't all afford a Tesla (although I eagerly await the Model 3 release), but we can certainly park like Tesla owners. Choose the parking space farther from your destination, and then enjoy the benefits of extra physical activity.

Use an activity tracker

Activity trackers are one of the most powerful tools for fighting back against the conspiracy to keep us in our chairs or in front of our computers.

I encourage all my clients to use them to establish new healthy rituals. Activity trackers measure your physical activity objectively. Seeing your steps accumulate can motivate you to move more.

With an activity tracker, you don't have to rely on your intuition that "I think I did a good job moving today." The little device keeps you accountable. Nothing motivates you more to end your day with a walk than looking at your activity tracker and seeing that you're 2000 steps short of your goal today—especially if you were thinking about plopping on the couch instead.

Most activity trackers also let you easily connect with friends and compare your activity level to theirs. You can compete with them, or simply use it as an extra level of support and accountability.

Before you know it, the 15-minute walk that you didn't think you had the time for becomes an important part of your day.

If my co-worker takes 12,000 steps in a day, I want to shoot for 12,001, just so I can silently gloat. But that's just me!

I recommend that you get a tracker and have fun with it. Use it as a motivator to increase your awareness of your activity level and get you moving more.

Garmin, FitBit, Misfit and others all have very good versions with various bells and whistles. Do your research to find out which specific features you want. Make sure it's user-friendly so you'll actually use it, and use your tracker to connect with like-minded people either online or in real life.

Exercise with more intensity

Based on the evidence, it certainly seems reasonable that shorter, more challenging higher-intensity bouts of exercise can meaningfully improve your overall health.

Participants in the study above who performed sprint interval training (SIT) cycled at maximum 100% effort. However, it's important for the rest of us to ease into high-intensity training.

An inexpensive heart-rate monitor can help you gauge the intensity level of your exercise and estimate your maximum heart rate (in fact, activity trackers from Garmin and FitBit now come with a heart rate monitor function). That way there's no guessing about your training level.

It would be reasonable and safe to start at 70% of your maximum effort, and then increase to 80% or 90% over the course of a few weeks. That allows your body to adjust and helps you learn what each level feels like.

I often suggest that clients start with bicycling, either on a stationary bike or on the road, or on a rowing machine. It's a great way to ease into higher-intensity exercise, with less impact and less risk of injury than running or interval circuit training. If you are looking for more motivation, group spin classes can be a great way to get you excited and your heart rate moving!

As you add higher-intensity and strength training to your exercise, I recommend supervision by a trained fitness professional to help you avoid injury and get the best results. Lots of options are available, from personal trainers to boot camps to spin classes at your local recreation center to Pilates classes at the local Y. Find what fits into your life and take advantage of the qualified experience of others!

Ignore your scale for a month

Remember that health and fitness are your goals, not weight loss. When you focus on health, appropriate weight loss will follow.

Studies have shown that overweight individuals who met criteria for being "fit" had similar health benefits as those who were "normal weight."

Being skinny doesn't equal being healthy. There are plenty of out of shape, unhealthy skinny folks out there.

Being fit, on the other hand, generally does correlate with health. Once you start exercising regularly, you may notice that clothes fit differently. You feel better—yet your weight has not changed.

Don't get discouraged. Weight loss will occur in a healthy and sustainable manner.

For this reason, I recommend that you do not get on a scale until you are four weeks into your program.

Scales can distract you from your true purpose: improving your health. If you lost only a little weight, but were able to stop your diabetes medicines, your blood pressure returned to normal, and you reduced your inflammation, would you still be as concerned with your weight?

What if you lost quite a bit of weight, but still struggled with fitness and made no meaningful difference in your health? That's not the path to lifelong health.

Focus on making the lifestyle changes, being healthy and feeling well. That's how I define success.

Exercise anxieties

Exercise is boring!

I can already hear many of you saying "Exercise is boring! I can't stick with it if I am always bored!" It's very true. If you find exercise boring, you likely will not stay with it.

My suggestions in this book are general guidelines. In truth, the best form of exercise is the one you'll do. It's a trial-and-error process to find what works for you.

Some thrive with the coaching and energy in group exercise classes, spin classes, or other classes at your local gym or YMCA.

Others want to be on their own to help clear their mind as they exercise. Still others enjoy the chance to catch up with friends or significant others on a long walk. And others prefer games with friends, like basketball, soccer or tennis.

Find what works for you and then own it! The key is to make sure you start moving and that you keep moving.

I'm afraid I'll hurt myself

This is a real concern for many, especially those who have not exercised regularly in the past. I cannot emphasize enough the importance of posture and functional alignment exercises and building strength and balance. These are your weapons to prevent injury. See more about this in the injury prevention section below.

In addition, always start and progress new activities slowly.

I've seen it countless times. After years of not exercising, our bodies are very different than they were in our prime.

Yet our minds remember the workouts we used to be able to do. Call it ego, or the quest for endorphins, or something else. Our common sense takes a back seat and we try to relive the glory days and exercise like it was 1999. The next day is never a pretty sight, and that type of pace is never sustainable.

Remember, our goal is healthy activities over your entire lifetime, not just the next few weeks. Be smart. Go slow. Get strong.

I have diabetes. Am I at risk of hypoglycemia?

If you're on medication like injectable insulin or sulfonylureas that increases your insulin levels and lowers your blood glucose, exercise could mildly increase your risk of low blood sugars. Fortunately, there is an easy solution. Test your blood glucose before and after you exercise. Have a preselected snack ready in case it drops significantly. You can also talk to your doctor about adjusting your insulin or medication dose prior to exercise.

I see people all the time who want to raise a low blood sugar as quickly as possible, so they eat candy, drink juice, or consume some other food that's very high in added sugars. This is the equivalent of killing a fly with a machine gun, and it sends their sugar and insulin levels on a rollercoaster.

Why does your blood sugar fall during exercise? Because your body is utilizing your blood sugar for energy, not storing it as fat. Maintain a regular exercise schedule, and you'll soon be able to taper down or even stop your medications. Just don't counteract the beneficial effects of that exercise by loading up on high-sugar foods devoid of nutrients.

Apple slices or plain Greek yogurt with a handful of berries will all correct your blood sugar without causing the sugar and insulin rollercoaster caused by the "junk" alternatives.

I have a chronic illness

What if you suffer from chronic fatigue syndrome (CFS) or fibromyalgia (FM)? Sometimes it is all you can do to get out of bed, let alone get regular exercise.

Even when it's difficult, regular exercise is crucial for your overall health and for your underlying condition. While some of my specific tips may not apply in this setting, the general concepts still apply.

In the beginning, you may not feel like exercising. You may feel like it is worthless since you will "never" be able to get the "required" amount of exercise.

Start by changing your mindset. Any activity or movement is better than none!

They keys are to set reachable short-term goals and do something on most days.

Rest between repetitions: rest for twice as long as it took you to do the exercise, and then repeat.

Celebrate your short-term victories. The long-term results only come if you succeed in the short term.

Many with CFS or FM have not exercised for so long that they have become severely deconditioned. In this case, start with range-of-motion exercises, like arm circles, leg raises, and sit-to-stand repetitions. Consider consulting a physical therapist, since certain exercises may be best avoided for fibromyalgia and some other conditions.

Tap your support community for ideas as well. Others with the same conditions have faced the same challenges and can offer valuable advice.

And remember: when making meaningful lifestyle changes, things won't always go perfectly. It will be a constant journey with roadblocks—and recoveries.

Expect them. Prepare for them. You will not be perfect. But you can always recover.

I'm worried about injury

Exercising with purpose also means that we need to be purposeful about protecting ourselves from exercise-induced injuries.

The risk of injury increases when we start a new exercise routine, and it also increases as we age. Our sedentary daily routine only further increases that risk.

For example, many of us have what physical therapists call an "upper-crossed" and "lower-crossed" syndrome. These fancy terms explain what happens to our bodies when we slouch over a computer, a phone, or just sit too long.

Think about your alignment right now as you read this book! Our lower abdominal and butt muscles— "glutes"—turn off, our heads lean forward, and our shoulders hunch forward. We're left with a slouched posture, tight chest and neck muscles, and very weak glute, back and core muscles.

Our injury risk is substantial if we start strength training or a high-intensity interval training program with this posture.

The cure is to reverse the activities that force us into improper positions.

That means addressing your work ergonomics and being mindful of your posture when you're on the phone, in the car, in a waiting room, or any other time you find yourself falling into a slouch.

TIP ◗ Stick a note on your computer screen that says "Sit up, Stand up and Move!" Get up and walk for two minutes for every 30 that you sit. Even if you can't walk around during the day, simply standing up forces you to reset your posture.

When you sit back down, think about contracting your glutes and your lower abs, sit up tall, retract your shoulder blades, and let your head drift up.

You don't have to maintain that alignment for a whole hour. Just the action of doing it for a few seconds multiple times each day is a powerful way to teach your body proper functional alignment.

The following simple exercises strengthen and retrain your functional alignment muscles. They help "wake up" the neuromuscular connections between your brain and these neglected muscles, thus improving your ability to turn them on.

Exercise 1

- ⊙ Lie on the floor with the back of your head, your heels, your shoulders and your butt flat.
- ⊙ Breathe in a full breath to fill your chest.
- ⊙ Now, breathe out.

- As you exhale, push your lower back against the floor and pull your belly button back to your spine. Make sure your head, heels and shoulders remain on the floor.
- Hold this position for the duration of your breath.
- Then, relax as you inhale again.
- Do this 10 times.

Exercise 2

- While lying on the floor, contract both of your butt muscles.
- Hold for 5 seconds and release.
- Do this 10 times.
- Then, contract each side individually, hold for 5 seconds and release. This exercise can definitely feel a little awkward. We spend so much time sitting with our glutes turned off that our bodies need a simple reminder that we can control and contract these muscles at will.

Exercise 3

- Stand against a flat wall with your heels and the back of your head touching the wall. Stand tall, with the crown of your head reaching for the sky.
- Press your shoulder blades back against the wall while pulling your belly button back to your spine.

⊙ Keep checking in on our body. "Are my heels touching the wall? Are my shoulders back? Is my belly button pulled in? Is my head high?" This allows you the chance to readjust.

⊙ This exercise will likely be uncomfortable at first. As you continue practicing, you'll gradually lengthen the amount of time you can do it.

As you progress to your weightlifting and resistance exercises, turning on these functional alignment muscles and focusing on the posture cues you learned in the above exercises will help you maximize your results and prevent injuries.

Fitness for more advanced participants

The "Move with Purpose" fitness program outlined at the end of this chapter is directed primarily at those who are new to exercise or have been unsuccessful in maintaining an exercise program in the past.

If you already exercise or are in moderate to good physical condition, these additional tips may be more helpful.

Diversity is king

Diversify your physical activity so that you have moderate cardiovascular exercise, high-intensity interval training (HIIT), strength training and functional alignment exercises.

As a triathlete, I trained for hours in long-distance swimming, cycling and running. After completing the Ironman, I felt like I was in the best shape of my life and I felt like I had never been healthier. I couldn't have been more wrong.

Sure, I was in excellent cardiovascular condition.

But I had completely neglected resistance training and functional alignment. It didn't take long for injuries to set in and force me to stop competing.

Naturally, I decided to take up golf. You can guess what happened next.

Injuries, injuries and more injuries. My training had prepared my body to move forward in a straight line. When I asked it to do anything else, it simply broke down.

I've reversed the damage to my body by diversifying my workout routines to include ample strength training and functional alignment exercises.

I continue to do HIIT and moderate cardiovascular exercise, and I can now say that my body is physically the best it has ever been.

Don't assume that your training is spot-on because you can run a marathon. Diversify!

Make your HIIT count

The first two words of HIIT say it all. High intensity.

When done correctly, HIIT should be challenging. You should get that uncomfortable feeling in your stomach, the burn in your lungs, the exhaustion in your muscles. Then you should rest. And do it again!

Far too often, people do HIIT for the first five minutes of their training routine and then fall back to moderate intensity the rest of the time. Yet they still call it a HIIT day.

That's one of many reasons I love interval training programs like Orange Theory Fitness.

They make your training objective. Your heart rate is right up there on the screen for everyone to see. If you aren't in the orange or red zone, then you aren't at high intensity. Simple.

Throw in the coaches and the community, and all of a sudden you have more than enough motivation to turn it up a notch.

Look for this level of engagement and intensity for your HIIT workout, whether it is a spin class, a boot camp, or just going after it with a few friends. Turn it up a notch and make your HIIT count!

Active recovery

Just as high intensity is important on your HIIT days, low intensity is important on your recovery days.

That doesn't mean doing remote control curls on the couch.

It means walking your dog or with your spouse (depending on whose company you enjoy more at that moment). It means going for an easy spin on the bike. It means focusing on your functional alignment exercises.

Just as HIIT should be a challenge, active rest and moderate cardio should be more routine.

Continue to move your body

Don't sit the rest of the day just because you went hard during your workout and got your high intensity work done.

That makes you a sedentary exerciser. That's certainly better than not exercising at all, but not nearly as beneficial as exercising and remaining active.

Make it fun

Even those who are exercise enthusiasts still get bored from time to time. Our routines get stale, it's harder to motivate to get to the gym, we feel like we are in a rut.

The solution is keeping it fun and diverse. What this looks like is different for everyone, so ask yourself what would make it more fun for you.

Join a community or group training center like Orange Theory or local boot camp. Make it social by running or biking with a group of friends.

Find something to train for like a charity bike ride, a local 5K, or even better a Spartan Race. Join a basketball league for a season.

Whatever it is, make it different and make it fun.

CONCLUSION

Here's why I said earlier that lack of exercise is one of the easiest issues to correct:

You don't actually have to formally exercise to move your body and improve your health!

Think of all the opportunities you have to move more during the day.

Walk the dog for 15 minutes. Park further from your destination and walk the extra couple minutes. Take the stairs instead of escalators or elevators. Work in the garden.

No gym membership or change of clothes required.

The key is to just start.

Simply move your body more and you're already improving your health.

If you can get 150 minutes of moderate exercise per week, that's fantastic. More is even better.

But if you can't, don't worry. You can still benefit your health dramatically simply by being active.

And as you add more frequent, longer-lasting activities, or you boost the intensity level, you'll reap even greater benefits.

THE PLAN: MOVE WITH PURPOSE

Here's the core principle behind this plan:

hen you exercise with purpose and intensity three days each week, and use your activity tracker to make sure you're moving more the rest of the week, you really don't need formal exercise every single day in order to achieve better health and lower your risk of chronic diseases.

Week 1

⊙　Increase your daily activity: park farther away, take the stairs, walk every 30 minutes at work, start a gardening project, etc.

⊙ Get an activity tracker and determine your baseline activity level.

Week 2

⊙ Start exercising daily for at least 15 minutes. That's it. Just 15 minutes. Walk when you get up, before dinner, at lunch. Just 15 minutes.

⊙ Pay attention to how your daily exercise changes your activity monitor data

⊙ Begin daily functional alignment exercises.

Week 3

⊙ Set your goal on your activity monitor. Shoot for at least 8,000-12,000 steps per day, keeping in mind that more is better. Adjust your goal according to your baseline activity level.

⊙ Exercise 30 minutes three days per week.

⊙ Continue daily posture exercises.

Week 4

⊙ Pick two of your exercise days and substitute high-intensity interval training and strength training on those days.

⊙ Consider starting off with a trainer or a fitness program

⊙ Make sure you're still hitting your
activity monitor goals at least five
days per week. If not, formulate a
specific plan for achieving that goal.

For journal citations and more insight
into the Copenhagen Heart Study,
Leisure Time & Mortality Study,
and other research in this chapter,
visit the Book Resources Blog at
DrBretScher.com.

6: Manage Your Stress and Sleep

DO MORE, EARN MORE, BE MORE

Do you get as much sleep as you'd like? Is your life relatively free of stress? Don't worry, those were rhetorical questions.

For the overwhelming majority of Americans, the answers are a resounding NO! Our "do more, earn more, be more" society places nearly all of us under significant daily pressure, forcing us to live with more stress and less and less sleep.

That's a problem.

Numerous studies have shown that stress increases cortisol and adrenaline levels in our bodies, and harms our health over time. These stress hormones are important for a temporary "fight-or-flight" response, but they are actually harmful over the long term. They routinely increase blood pressure and inflammation markers, causing weight gain or resisting attempts to lose weight, and decreasing your overall well-being.

Here's the shocker, though: these studies also discovered that the effect of stress on your health is *under your control*. Stress itself isn't the problem.

It's how our bodies react to the stress. And that can be under our control!

People who view stress as bad, or negative, are likelier to experience harmful health effects. People who don't see stress as negative tend to avoid those harmful effects.

This is powerful research, because it once again shows that we are masters of our destiny. We can't eliminate all stress from our lives. That just isn't practical. Yet we can drastically reduce the harmful effects of our stressful and busy lifestyles with the right tools and the right mindset.

The answer is to train your body to handle stress so that you don't have an aggressive physiological response to the stress.

How can we do that? It starts with being mindful.

THE EVIDENCE FOR MINDFULNESS

Mindful meditation is the ultimate stress-buster.

It won't make your boss stop yelling at you. It won't make that deadline go away. But it will change how your body reacts to the unavoidable stressors in your life.

Mindfulness simply means that we acknowledge our thoughts and feelings without judging them. We don't need to categorize our feelings as good or bad, right or wrong. Instead, we can simply note how we feel in the present moment, without connecting it to a past feeling or future fear.

Is that too simple to have a profound impact on our health? No way!

Studies have shown that practicing mindful meditation, instead of judgment, can improve your immune function, reduce overly emotional reactions, and improve your overall wellbeing.

Many people are shocked when they first hear that mindfulness can even change the physical structure of your brain. Yet it's true. A Harvard study showed that regular mindful practice can actually change the anatomy of your brain, thus leading to improved emotional functions.

These studies also help explain why mindfulness has become so popular in recent years: it's a very powerful, and easily usable, tool for dealing with stressful situations.

NEXT STEPS

Modify your stress management mindset

What do you think of when you hear the words "mindfulness" and "meditation"?

Do you picture monks in a remote mountain village, sworn to silence, sitting for hours trying to free their minds of all thoughts, and then levitating above the ground?

Or do you think of Apple founder Steve Jobs, one of the most creative and innovative humans ever to start a business—and a committed practitioner of mindful meditation?

Often, people with a fixed mindset hear "meditation" or "mindfulness" and think, "Are you kidding? No way will this lower my stress." Sometimes they worry about looking silly, or think that they won't be able to do it "right" for some reason. Sometimes they fear that it might even compromise their own beliefs.

I encourage you to throw away these preconceptions about mindful meditation. Instead, practice a growth mindset and keep yourself open to the possibilities as you learn more.

Meditation was once felt to be only for deeply pious individuals who dedicated their life to mindfulness. Today, it is a mainstream practice and a near-requirement for creativity, innovation and productivity. As Mr. Jobs pointed out, meditation calms a mind that's constantly swerving from one thought to another, from one anxiety to another. Once your mind slows down, your imagination and resourcefulness start to resurface. That's when you can achieve more than you ever thought possible.

I can't promise that a regular mindfulness meditation practice will make you as brilliant and creative as Steve Jobs. I *can* promise that it will help you temper your body's reaction to stress, help you think more clearly, feel more balanced, and help unleash your true potential.

I know what you're thinking. "What difference does it make if I meditate for 10 minutes and then a few minutes later I'm sitting in traffic yelling at the car next to me?"

Meditation is like exercise. If you exercise today, you may feel great. The blood is flowing and the endorphins are pumping. But if you don't exercise again for two months, you won't retain the benefits from that single week of exercising. On the other hand, if you exercise four days every week, week in and week out, you'll see dramatic short *and* long-term benefits. Your strength and fitness gains will improve every minute of every day of your life, not just the minutes you spend exercising.

The same applies to your mindful meditation practice. Your daily mindful meditation "trains" your brain to react differently in stressful situations. With practice, your mind and body will learn to stop overreacting to stress and to restore a sense of relaxation.

Then, when that inevitable stress comes into your life, *you* will be the one who can control your body's reaction. You won't experience that cortisol and adrenaline spike that I mentioned earlier. You won't get the blood pressure spike. And you won't have chronic inflammation from chronic stress reactions. All because you prepared for that moment with a regular mindful practice.

Four steps to mindful meditation

Starting your mindful meditation practice is easy to do, and easy to fit into your schedule.

Start with just five minutes, and work your way up to 10, 15 or even 20 minutes.

Here's a simple four-step process to get you going:

Step 1

- ⊙ Sit comfortably in a quiet place with few distractions.
- ⊙ You don't need to sit cross-legged or hold your fingers in a specific position. You don't have to sit on the floor.
- ⊙ Just be comfortable.

Step 2

- ⊙ Close your eyes and notice your thoughts.

- ⊙ Don't try to stop or control these thoughts. Just observe them, like a third-party observer looking in from the outside.

Step 3

- ⊙ Breathe. Focusing on your breath is central to mindfulness.

- ⊙ Feel your breath as it comes in and out through your nose.

- ⊙ As you focus on your breath, more thoughts will come in to interrupt your focus, and that's okay.

- ⊙ Don't judge your thoughts and don't try to control them. Simply observe and acknowledge them.

- ⊙ Then move your focus back to your breath.

Step 4

- ⊙ Become aware of how your body feels.

- ⊙ Notice the heaviness of your head, the feeling of your hands resting on your legs or in your lap, your feet touching the ground, the air moving in and out of your nose as you breath.

And that's it. Those are the basics of being mindful. It may feel foreign at first, but like any new skill, you become more adept the more you practice it.

Be in the present, focus on your breathing, and allow the world to continue without reacting to it. Allow your thoughts to come and go without trying to control them, chase them away, or react to them.

Here are more tips that will help you succeed in this new habit:

- ⊙ Meditate as soon as you wake up. Don't wait for a stressful situation to remind you to meditate. Make it part of your daily routine and stick to a schedule. It's otherwise too easy to let it slide.

- ⊙ Use a timer to keep your brain from wandering to questions like "Shouldn't I be done already?" With a timer, you'll know when time is up.

- ⊙ Start with 5 minutes. Increase it to 10 minutes after the first week.

- ⊙ Consider an online app like Headspace or local meditation classes when you first get started. Eventually you'll feel comfortable meditating on your own. Meanwhile, having someone guide you is invaluable.

- ⊙ Celebrate every mindfulness practice, even if you felt that you were more distracted today. It's all part of the learning process. Simply taking the time to sit and practice mindfulness is a victory in itself.

There's no right or wrong way to practice meditation, and there are no good or bad meditation sessions. Stick with it and enjoy the process.

Physically active meditations

If you try the seated approach for two weeks and it just doesn't work for you, consider one of these alternatives:

- ⊙ Tai chi
- ⊙ Yoga
- ⊙ Mindful walking

Like seated meditation, these methods focus on your breathing and on observing how your body feels.

Allow thoughts to come and go without addressing them or reacting to them. Observe how your body feels and moves as you perform the tai chi postures, yoga poses, or simply walk with intention. Focus on the rhythm of your breathing as air moves in and out.

These practices offer benefits that are similar to seated meditation, although the anatomical and physiological benefits haven't been as fully researched.

One of my clients who finds it a challenge to sit still for more than two minutes swears by her mindful dog walks.

She focuses on her dog's ears as they flop up and down. This focus helps her remain in the present, avoid distractions, and remain mindful. The key is finding the practice that works for you.

Make every day mindful

Remind yourself every day that "I am in control of my stress. I am in control of my reactions." Simply saying those sentences as part of a daily affirmation helps you reframe your mindset and be more open to a mindful practice.

TIP ⊙ Next time a stressor confronts you, take stock of your body's response. Where did you feel the stress? Did you clench your teeth? Your hands? Did your heart speed up or did you feel a little nauseous?

Take note of your response and remember it the next time you encounter stress. Don't fall back into your prior reactions. Instead, make your immediate response simply breathing, just as you do in your daily mindfulness practice.

Don't think, don't act, don't react. Just breathe. Feel the air come in and out of your body. Feel the weight of your body as your shoulders sink and your jaw relaxes.

Use those breaths and body awareness to remind yourself that you are in control of your reaction. Even if you can't control the stress, you can control your body.

You'll also want to look for opportunities to incorporate your mindfulness habit into your daily activities. Not only does this help you be more mindful, it also helps you become more grateful for what you have and what it took to get to you.

Start with your morning cup of coffee or tea. Take three deep breaths as you drink it, and appreciate the smell, the warmth, and the taste.

Then, when you sit down to eat, be present with your meal.

Notice the colors of the food.

Close your eyes and appreciate the smells.

Take your first bite and appreciate the taste.

Envision the process your food took to reach your plate—the soil and sun that helped it grow, the farmer who planted it, the worker who packed it, the person who cut it up and cooked it.

Wait, don't stop yet!

Take three deep breaths as you're brushing your teeth, washing the dishes, or my personal favorite, stopped at the traffic light.

Focus on the air coming in and out of your nose and notice the sensations all around you.

Don't think about all that you have to do today. You'll have plenty of time to think about that later.

Take the moment to be in the present and let your mind be at peace. Your mind, your body and your health will thank you for it.

Mindful Traffic Jams

I hate traffic. I hate feeling like I'm stuck and can't get where I want to go. I used to be the guy squeezing the steering wheel until my knuckles were white. Once I realized the effect this was having on my body, I knew I needed a solution. I didn't realize just how easy that solution was!

Now when I'm stuck in traffic, I think to myself, "This is the perfect opportunity to practice my mindfulness." Instead of strangling the steering wheel, I take three deep breaths (eyes open for this mindful exercise!) and feel the air as it comes

YOUR BEST HEALTH EVER!

in and goes out. I take stock of how my body
is feeling and I focus on my present moment.
Suddenly, traffic doesn't seem so bad and my
body's reaction becomes dramatically different.

And best of all, I'm not a stressed-out mess when I
get home. Instead, I'm relaxed, calm and ready to
enjoy the wonderful chaos that confronts me as I
open the front door!

• •

THE RECIPE FOR BETTER SLEEP

YAWN.....

We all need more sleep, right?

You've heard it hundreds, maybe thousands, of
times. "Get more sleep for better health."

Yet a huge gap exists between the recommendation
and our actions.

For many of us, our lives are so over-busy, over-
scheduled, and over-stressed that sleep is the last
item on our priority list. And even when we try to
get more sleep, many things can prevent that from
happening.

We need a road map for overcoming these
obstacles.

THE EVIDENCE FOR SLEEP

The scientific literature is saturated with evidence
that sleep is important for health.

Here's just a partial list of the potential harms from poor sleep:

- Depression
- Anxiety
- Weight gain
- Diabetes
- Hypertension
- Coronary artery disease
- Strokes
- Poor job performance
- Poor athletic performance
- More car accidents

Making the problem even worse, many people with inadequate sleep actually feel like they're doing just fine. But they're wrong.

A fascinating 2003 study in the journal *Sleep* showed that people who got no more than six hours of daily sleep for 10 consecutive days suffered almost the same cognitive and physical declines as people who were completely deprived of sleep for three whole days.

The amazing part is that the first group had no idea how bad their performance was. They did not feel tired. They felt they were thinking clearly and performing well on all the required tests. That makes it even more dangerous! To perform so poorly and not even realize it is a recipe for disaster.

At least those who were deprived of sleep for three whole days knew they were exhausted. If their everyday lives were this sleep-deprived, they would likely recognize the problem and could then make appropriate changes. The same cannot be said for the group who got less than 6 hours of sleep per night. They didn't perceive any problems and would probably be unlikely to make any changes.

Yet another incredible study examined the sleep patterns of traditional hunter-gatherer tribes. Sleep problems were so rare in these cultures that the three tribes studied did not even have words for sleep problems like insomnia in their language.

The study showed that they averaged 7.5–8 hours in bed each night. They followed a consistent sleep-wake schedule, thus maintaining a stable daily rhythm. Combined with their computer-free, phone-free, distraction-free society, it's no wonder they had no concept of sleep problems. Industrialized society can learn valuable lessons from their life habits!

Last, numerous studies have shown that poor sleep habits result in an inability to lose weight due to increased hunger, increased snacking, and poor food choices.

That's because inadequate sleep affects hormones that influence hunger and appetite. Ghrelin, the "hunger hormone," signals to your body that you're hungry and need to eat. The hormone leptin has the opposite effect, and signals that you're full and don't need to eat. Poor sleep causes spikes in ghrelin, and suppresses leptin. Add this to the rise in cortisol and it's no wonder that lack of sleep is directly linked to weight gain.

Leptin, ghrelin and cortisol are major reasons for why we feel hungry and snack more when we're sleep deprived. Plus, since lack of sleep reduces our mental clarity and our ability to control our emotions, we tend to react impulsively when we feel hungry. Impulse decisions rarely end in a well-balanced meal of veggies with healthy fats and proteins. More often, the result is standing in front of the freezer, door open, eating Ben and Jerry's right from the carton with no end in sight.

We've all been there. Fortunately, we all get another chance the very next day to be more mindful about our actions and be better. A good night's sleep will certainly help!

Wasted time or regenerative time?

Some people argue that "Sleep is a waste of time. It's unproductive time I could spend accomplishing things."

This couldn't be further from the truth. The normal human sleep cycle consists of five phases: Stages 1, 2, 3, 4 and REM (rapid eye movement) sleep. Without adequate time in each stage of sleep, the body can't perform its essential "reboot" functions.

For example, your body literally restores itself during "restorative sleep," which is the combination of Stage 3 sleep and REM sleep.

During Stage 3 sleep, also known as "deep sleep" or "delta wave sleep," your body heals and restores physical energy. REM sleep improves learning, memory and concentration. Without ample time in these stages, your body misses prime opportunities to become more productive the next day.

In addition, alcohol and sleep medications can disrupt the balance of sleep stages, thus resulting in less restorative sleep.

Part of the importance of maintaining a steady sleep schedule is that it allows your body to cycle through the stages of sleep consistently, ensuring that you get adequate time in the deep and restorative stages.

NEXT STEPS

Modify your sleep mindset

Many of us surrendered to a fixed mindset about sleep years ago. We resigned ourselves to inadequate sleep, or poor quality sleep. We feel like we've tried everything. We label ourselves as "insomniacs" or just "poor sleepers" and now, simply accept our fate. If we raise the issue with our doctor, what follows next is usually a series of prescriptions for potentially addictive sleeping pills.

Popular news sources estimate that prescriptions for sleeping medications have increased more than 50% since 2008. That's a huge increase! And the biggest problem is that those drugs don't actually "fix" anything. We may feel that they help us sleep, but they're still a far cry from achieving the same result naturally.

As with many things in medicine, prescription drugs are just short-term band-aids. They treat the symptom without addressing the underlying cause. They also distort the stages of sleep, so that you miss out on the full restorative power of natural sleep, and they also come with the risk of dependence, rebound insomnia, and short-term memory loss.

What if we could change our mindsets?

Instead of resigning ourselves to poor sleep, what if we believed that our ability to sleep well was within our control?

To start changing your mindset, consider questions like these:

- ⊙ What if I could improve my sleep habits?

- ⊙ What if I were able to feel more energetic, think more clearly, and just feel better during the day?

Simply asking these questions helps us transition to a growth mindset and helps us believe more and better sleep is possible.

Now, visualize your goal of sleeping soundly through the night and waking up refreshed, and consider these questions:

- ⊙ How do you feel?

- ⊙ How calm and relaxed is your mind?

Now go one step further. Visualize the habits that helped you achieve that goal.

- ⊙ What time did you go to sleep?

- ⊙ What were you doing right before you went to sleep?

- ⊙ What were you thinking about as you got into bed?

- ⊙ What did your bedroom look, feel, and sound like?

These are the habits we need to develop to become better sleepers.

Create your sleep retreat

Give yourself the gift of making your bedroom a welcoming, enjoyable and peaceful sleep retreat.

Your bedroom is for sleeping, so your goal is to make it as inviting for sleep as you possibly can.

Change your mind set about your room to acknowledge that it is now a peaceful sleep retreat. Make this a daily affirmation statement. As you approach your room, say out loud, "I am entering my peaceful sleep retreat. The concerns of the day are over and can be addressed tomorrow. Now it is time for sleep."

The more you repeat that simple phrase, the more your body will understand it to be true and start to physiologically prepare for sleep (try it, it works!).

Choose whatever decor will make you feel more at home and more relaxed. Make it visually pleasing by displaying relaxing and enjoyable art, photos of your family, or pictures of the beach. You can use a very mild scent to signal the separation between your sleep retreat and the rest of the house. You can also use light bulbs with a softer light.

When you walk into your bedroom, you want to feel that the day has melted away, your concerns have all been addressed, and there is nothing left to do other than to sleep.

One of my favorite sleep medicine physicians likes to say that you don't have insomnia if you have all the lights on in the bedroom, you're watching "Psycho" in bed on your iPad, and you suddenly decide it's time to go to sleep.

Of course you won't be able to sleep! Control your surroundings first before labeling yourself as an insomniac.

A peaceful sleep retreat, by definition, is empty of the technological devices that turn on your brain and increase alertness. No televisions, smartphones, tablets, or laptops.

Do your work, your reading, and your Facebook and Twitter updates in another space *before* you enter your bedroom. Do your thinking, your planning, and even your journaling somewhere else.

Do not do these activities in your bedroom.

Think about all that you need to do *before* you enter your bedroom.

Then, choose a time when you can address these matters more fully.

"I can address this on my lunch break from work tomorrow."

"I can pick up the toys and clean the dishes after the kids get to school tomorrow."

Without a concrete time to address them, your concerns will likely linger in your brain and disrupt your ability to peacefully drift off to sleep. However, assigning a specific time to address these issues allows your brain to have closure for the night. You can let go of the feeling that there are unanswered questions to address.

What if a thought pops into your head after you're tucked into bed? Once work-related thoughts or planning creep into the bedroom, it's like turning on a faucet. More thoughts will quickly follow! The ultimate goal is to turn that faucet off, but even turning it down is very beneficial.

You have two realistic choices.

You could practice your mindfulness. Let the thought come and go, acknowledge it but do not react to it. Focus on being in the present in your sleep retreat.

Or, keep a notepad by the bed. Write down your thought, choose a time to address more fully, and then go back to bed.

The key is to have closure. Whether it's physical, like writing it down, or mental, like your mindfulness practice, closure is what turns off the faucet of thoughts and helps you get back to your peaceful retreat. You can train your mind to expect this and react this way. You may not perfect this in one night, but over time it becomes second nature.

Reduce screen time

The most important sleep hygiene habit for most people is reducing time spent in front of computers, smartphones, tablets and e-readers.

 In the old days, a television was the only "screen" we had in our bedrooms. The television was against the wall opposite the bed, far away from our faces. That wasn't ideal for sleep, but it was certainly better than today's screens which are usually mere inches from our faces.

The blue light from laptops, smartphones and tablets disrupts our natural 24-hour physical, mental and behavior cycles, the "circadian rhythm" of our bodies. It also disrupts melatonin and other sleep hormones.

This disruption resets our brain's internal clock and erroneously tells our brains to stay alert, that it's not time for sleep yet. We keep triggering the cascade of events that keeps us functioning at a high level. Then we expect to fall asleep immediately as soon as we turn the screen off. Unfortunately our brains don't have the same "off" switch that our devices have. The result: poor-quality sleep.

The best solution to this problem is a simple one: cut out screens at least one hour before bed.

Many clients will ask, "If I can't use my computer or phone, what should I do?"

I feel a little sad when I get that question. I usually suggest using an old-fashioned pen and paper for journaling, or reading a book made of actual paper—not an e-book!

You can also practice your mindful meditation. You can use this time without screens to connect with your family members in a more personal and humane way, talking, playing card games or board games, or reading stories together.

One of my clients started doing crossword puzzles with her spouse. Not only was this a great screen-free activity, it helped build a new connection with her spouse and grew her vocabulary immensely!

If you have children, use this as an opportunity to set an example for them. Make a ritual of purposely turning off your devices. Talk about how unplugging and unwinding is a priority, and preparing for sleep is likewise a priority

If you absolutely cannot go without devices prior to the time you enter your sleep retreat—remember, the device does *not* come into your bedroom!—try orange-tinted glasses. These can help mitigate the harmful effects of blue light.

Many companies make these, and BluBlockers seems to be a popular brand. Various apps are also available which can lower blue light emissions. These strategies help somewhat, but are not completely effective. The most effective strategy is simply to avoid devices for the hour prior to bedtime.

Daily habits of successful sleepers

These tips will improve your chances of getting proper, restorative sleep. Most of these suggestions cost nothing and are easy to implement.

Maintain a consistent schedule

Going to bed and waking up at the same time every day has been scientifically shown to improve sleep quality by allowing consistent, deep, restorative sleep. The hunter-gatherer societies don't even have a word for insomnia. They all tend to have extraordinarily consistent sleep schedules. Consistency trains your body to know when it's time to prepare for sleep.

Go to sleep at the right time

The actual time you go to bed does matter. I like the saying: "An hour before midnight is worth two after midnight." Given our natural sleep-wake patterns, try to go to bed earlier, around 10 p.m., for example. The light-dark cycle of our day naturally primes our bodies to sleep earlier.

Practice meditation

In one study, people who practiced mindfulness had better sleep, less depression and less fatigue than those who simply received general sleep hygiene education. Even 10 minutes of mindfulness meditation achieves proven results.

Avoid caffeine in the afternoon and evening

Caffeine is a stimulant that can keep you from falling asleep.

Even people who say caffeine doesn't keep them awake in fact have reduced sleep quality compared with those who don't consume caffeine. Caffeine can stimulate our bodies for five to ten hours! You can still have your cup in the morning, but get rid of the afternoon caffeine to ensure better sleep.

Limit alcohol

Although alcohol may make you feel sleepy, it can dramatically alter the stages of sleep and prevent you from getting fully restorative sleep.

Limit liquids

The more you drink, the more likely you are to wake up to urinate.

That gives your brain a chance to wake up and start spinning, reducing your chances of going back to sleep. Try to stop drinking after 7 p.m., especially if you are a man with an enlarged prostate.

Get sunlight during the day

Studies in contemporary hunter-gatherer societies have highlighted the importance of daytime light exposure. Sunlight helps your body's natural rhythms stay in sync with proper sleep-wake patterns. This may also help with your vitamin D levels, which are linked to better sleep quality.

Exercise during the day

Exercise helps calibrate your internal clock and your body's hormones and often increases your exposure to sunlight. Just make sure you finish exercising at least one hour before going to bed.

Keep your room cool

Studies have shown that the ideal temperature for your bedroom is between 60-68 degrees. This allows your body to relax more deeply and get into deeper sleep faster.

Maintain a very dark room for sleeping

Use blackout shades. Cover your clocks, or keep them more than 3 feet away from your head). Use low wattage yellow, orange or red lights, not standard white lights. Colored lights stimulate your brain less, reducing the chance that it will think it's daytime.

Use your bed for sleeping and intimacy only

No computers, tablets, smartphones, televisions, books or journals.

Journal before bed

Getting your thoughts on paper helps clear your mind, so that your brain isn't ruminating on them instead of letting you fall asleep. Just remember to do it in another room!

Take magnesium supplements

Magnesium doses between 400 and 1000 milligrams can help you fall asleep and stay asleep. The best-absorbed magnesium supplements are in the form of glycinate, citrate, or malate. Alternatively, you can also take a warm Epson salt (magnesium sulfate) bath, and get your dose through skin absorption. A warm bath before bed can also help relax your mind and serve as a consistent reminder that it's time to let go of the day and prepare for sleep.

Take melatonin supplements when appropriate

Short-term use of melatonin doses between 1 – 3 milligrams can help improve sleep during travel or other temporary sleep cycle disruptions. Don't take it long-term, because it can disrupt your brain's natural production of melatonin.

Get checked for sleep apnea

Sleep apnea is most common among overweight people and those who drink alcohol or take sedatives. You doctor can order a simple home screening test for this very common cause of poor sleep. Fortunately, sleep apnea frequently can be treated with the same lifestyle interventions noted throughout this book.

Once you understand the importance of restorative sleep, and prioritize sleep as a pillar of your health, the above list becomes an easy "to do" list. If you could increase your productivity, improve your health, and have more energy with these simple lifestyle interventions, wouldn't you want to do it? I know I do!

CONCLUSION

Stress reduction is an example of a powerful health intervention that doesn't require a prescription or a pill.

We can't always control the stress that comes into our lives—yet with practice, we can control the way we react to that stress. A consistent mindful practice retrains our bodies to reduce our stress hormone release, minimizing its detrimental health effects.

It's also time for all of us to give sleep the priority it deserves.

The pressures of our modern society can make that seem daunting. Yet you can gain control of your sleep schedule with the tips in this chapter. You can train your body to get the restorative and beneficial sleep that you deserve every day. When you do, you'll see improvements in your daily life you never thought were possible.

THE PLAN: MANAGE YOUR STRESS & SLEEP

Week 1

- ⊙ Practice becoming mindful during your daily activities. Practice being in the present.

- ⊙ Pay attention to the stressors in your daily life and notice how you respond to stress. Take note. Do you clench your teeth or your fists? Do you feel an uneasy sensation in your stomach?

⊙ Start to breathe first, before you respond, and see how it changes your physical response to the stressor.

Week 2

⊙ Create your welcoming and peaceful sleep retreat.

⊙ Create pleasing sensations with pictures, smells or sounds.

⊙ Keep your room cool and completely dark.

⊙ Remove activities from the bedroom.

⊙ Eliminate screen time one-hour before bedtime.

⊙ Set a consistent sleep schedule.

⊙ Repeat your positive statement that your bedroom is your peaceful sleep retreat.

Week 3

⊙ Start sitting for a five-minute meditation session.

⊙ Make this a consistent schedule so that you sit at the same time every day. You can do it when you wake up, when you're about to go to sleep, during your lunch break, or anytime that's quiet.

⊙ Don't wait for a crazy moment when you need to calm yourself down. Meditation is preventive and mind-forming, not crisis management. Remember, it is not about doing it

right or wrong. The process is the
goal.

Week 4

- ⊙ Increase your meditation sessions
  to 10 minutes and include mindful
  practices in your daily activities.

- ⊙ Focus on your breathing during work,
  during your walks, and especially
  during times of stress or struggle.

- ⊙ Focus on being present and
  breathing.

For journal citations and more insight
into the studies of sleep, stress,
meditation, brain function, hunter-
gatherer lifestyles and other research
from this chapter, visit the Book
Resources Blog at DrBretScher.com.

7: Build Your Support Community

Have you ever tried to make big changes in your life all by yourself? Without involving friends or loved ones? It's hard! It's much easier to make big changes when you surround yourself with people who support you. That's why building a community is an integral part of sustaining healthy life habits.

Social support also has a dramatic effect on our mindset. Having others to support us helps reframe negative experiences toward the positive, and keeps us from dwelling in a negative mindset.

THE EVIDENCE FOR COMMUNITY

The leading research in this field began in 1938 and is still underway over 75 years later! The purpose of this study is to identify the attributes linked to greater well-being and a happier life. Researchers are following a group of about 300 male Harvard students and their families, and another group of about 500 men and their families from a poor, uneducated section of Boston.

After following them for decades, researchers have found that the best predictor of happiness and well-being is the quality of relationships with friends and spouses—not how much money they make, what car they drive, or what job they have.

Hundreds of other studies have reached similar conclusions, and have shown that people who maintain close social relationships are happier, less depressed, and feel a greater sense of purpose. These researchers have suggested numerous mechanisms that may link stronger social relationships to greater well-being.

One theory is that social ties hold us accountable for our actions, so we're less likely to do risky things like smoke tobacco or abuse alcohol and drugs. Another theory is that when we live with responsibility for others, like a spouse or children, we're more likely to find a deeper purpose for living well that motivates us to make better health choices. It's part of "finding our purpose," as I discussed in chapter 3.

Last, studies have shown that deeper social connections actually have a physiological effect on our bodies. It can improve our immune, endocrine and cardiovascular function, just to name a few. The opposite is also true. Stressful and negative social interactions, like a failing marriage, can increase stress response, decrease immune and endocrine function, and lead to a negative well-being.

NEXT STEPS

Modify your mindset

There's a difference between wanting to change and actually changing.

In fact, there's a famous model of healthy behavior change called the "transtheoretical model," developed in 1997 by Prochaska and Velicer. Their research found that people who make healthy changes go through five distinct stages.

In each stage, our mindset is distinctly different. In the "precontemplation" stage, for instance, we're not even thinking about making a change. In later stages, we haven't made the change—but we're seriously thinking about it. For example, we might read about the pros and cons of different ways of eating, or investigate membership costs at a gym.

As you move through each stage, you become more invested in the new behavior. Eventually, you've become that person who's ready to set foot along the course to a healthier you.

At first, your steps are uncertain. You may feel like you're walking in the dark, and you're not sure exactly where you're going. That's normal. Others like you are going through the same process.

That's why, in this stage, it's important to surround yourself with others who understand and support your behavior change.

Build your own community

Friends and family are usually the easiest place to start building your community. But don't be surprised if some are not as willing to help as you may have thought.

Some may be skeptical, or jealous. Some may say they will support you but end up being consistently negative.

The key is to find those who will support you and be positive, yet will still be honest and critical when necessary. Surround yourself with people who make you want to succeed. Those who make you feel better about yourself yet still keep you accountable.

Look to your workplace

Who do you spend the most time with during the day? For many it is your co-workers. Who better to enroll in your community than those you spend 8 hours a day with, sitting for long hours and fighting the urge to snack from the office candy jar?

Having your community members at work makes it that much easier to remember to get up and move on a regular basis, to bring your own healthy lunch from home, to go for a walk on your break, and, of course to stay away from the candy jar!

In addition, many employers offer wellness programs and provide extensive onsite resources to help you maintain your healthy lifestyle. Common options range from group exercise classes to walking clubs, interdepartmental wellness challenges and many other programs that help you surround yourself with a community of like-minded individuals. You may even get a benefit on your health insurance for participating in these programs!

If such groups don't already exist, you may find that your employer is happy to help you start one.

Enlist your healthcare providers

Ideally, your healthcare providers will become an integral part of your support community. Don't be shy. Be upfront with your providers, discuss your goals with them and explain your road map for achieving those goals.

Not only will they support you, they may be able to provide additional resources or connect you with others on a similar path, thus helping to build your support community further.

Once they are in your inner circle of supporters, your healthcare practitioners may be more proactive in helping you get off your medications, or helping you promote health as more than just the absence of disease. You will never know If you don't reach out to them!

Reach out locally

If you look hard enough, you can find a community to join right in your neighborhood.

Municipal recreation departments often offer free or inexpensive classes centered around a variety of healthy lifestyle habits, including sports and exercise, healthy eating and cooking, stress management and more. Local recreation centers often provide a pool, gym, and meeting place for those interested in a healthy lifestyle.

Many large churches and temples provide both facilities and classes for their members. It's an excellent way to meet people who share an interest in your healthy lifestyle goals.

Meetup.com is another useful resource for creating or locating groups whose members have similar interests, and NextDoor.com helps you connect to people in your neighborhood. For example, I can find my neighborhood's walking group schedule in our NextDoor forum.

Join an online community

We tend to develop deeper relationships in person, so the online community is not meant to replace the stronger bonds with your friends and family. There is, however, a wealth of chat rooms, Facebook groups, and support sites online that can help you on your journey.

Pick the ones that connect best with you to add an extra layer of support to your growing social community. Get out there and build those social bonds!

If the online community is large enough, some members will be at a similar point in their journey. Others will be farther along. Reach out for support, ideas and constructive criticism to help you overcome challenges and reinforce the steps you're taking. You'll create rewarding friendships with a strong mutual bond based on shared interests.

Celebrate as a community

Share your successes with your community, whether it's your friends, family or an online group. Nothing feels as good as an "attaboy" from those who know you best.

Your mom may not understand just how far you've come. Your coworkers may never notice that you always choose the most distant parking spot.

But the people who support your journey, like the neighbor who speed-walks with you on the weekend, will recognize your accomplishment and celebrate it with you.

Remember to cheer on your community, too. You may feel that you're still a work in progress—yet your praise is priceless for those on the journey with you.

CONCLUSION

Ultimately, the challenge is individual. Nobody can eat better, exercise, or manage your stress for you. But those who have walked the same path know what you're going through. They can remind you that there's a light at the end of the tunnel. And surrounding yourself with those who want to help you pays substantial dividends in the long run.

The research is clear: maintaining strong connections to other people who support us is a vital pillar for our overall health. It leads to increased happiness, a greater sense of purpose, and makes our healthy lifestyle habits easier to maintain long-term.

One of the most important aspects of community is the sense of shared ownership of challenges. Whether it's a local group or an online community, the principle is the same: members facing similar hurdles succeed when they combine their efforts.

And make sure you remember to celebrate your community! They're there to cheer your victories, and help support you when you slip. Count on them to be honest and hold you accountable, without tearing you down.

Don't be surprised when one day—sooner than you think—someone in your community starts looking to you for insight.

THE PLAN: BUILD YOUR SUPPORT COMMUNITY

Week 1

- ⊙ Talk about your goals with your friends and loved ones.

- ⊙ Gauge their responses. Are they supportive, or dubious? Constructive, or critical?

- ⊙ Use this feedback to help you decide who to include in your community, and enroll at least two people the first week

Week 2

- ⊙ Expand your community to your workplace and your local neighborhood

- ⊙ Communicate your goals with your healthcare providers and explore what support they may provide.

Week 3

- ⊙ Explore online communities, through activity trackers, social media sites, message forums and elsewhere to expand your reach, increase learning opportunities, and explore new aspects of your health journey.

Week 4

⊙ Celebrate as a community. Have a formal celebration event and define the successes you are choosing to celebrate. Don't forget, you are celebrating your support community as much as they are celebrating your successes.

For journal citations and more insight into the studies of community, peer support and other research from this chapter, visit the Book Resources Blog at DrBretScher.com.

8: Re-Examine Your Healthcare

Would you rather fix an underlying problem, or would you rather mask a symptom while allowing the underlying problem to fester?

When asked like this, the answer seems obvious. So why has our healthcare system evolved to focus more on prescription medications that may improve symptoms but often don't resolve the underlying cause?

In a way, it makes sense. This can be a very rewarding system for both doctor and patient. You come into the doctor's office with heartburn. The doctor writes a prescription for a proton pump inhibitor (PPI) that reduces stomach acid. Within a few hours, your symptoms are gone. You're happy and feel better, and the doctor justifiably feels successful for having helped you.

At your next visit, your lab tests show your "bad" cholesterol is elevated. Your doctor prescribes a statin drug. On the next test, your "bad" number is lower.

Again, everyone's happy in a short amount of time.

So what's the problem with this approach?

First, it assumes that relieving the immediate symptom or improving the lab result means that we've solved the underlying problem and produced lasting improvements in your health.

Second, it assumes that the medications given for the problem are safe and effective for long-term use.

As a cardiologist, however, I can tell you that the symptom-based, prescription-based approach frequently does not address the underlying problem.

Why are your cholesterol numbers elevated? And is that even a concern?

Why are you experiencing frequent heartburn?

There has to be an underlying reason.

If you keep banging your knee on your coffee table, do you become an expert at taking care of your own wounds, or do you move the coffee table?

If we control your immediate symptoms and consider ourselves done, are we leaving unresolved an underlying condition that over time may lead to more serious health problems?

All too often the answer is a resounding yes!

We should therefore ask ourselves:

Is there something else we can do, without medications, to eradicate the underlying problem?

Again, the answer is usually yes!

But we'll never find out unless we ask the question.

BE YOUR BEST HEALTH ADVOCATE

In this chapter, I want to empower you to understand the difference between treating symptoms and treating the underlying condition.

I want you to realize that we can achieve amazing health benefits through purposeful lifestyle interventions. In fact, these benefits are frequently better than those we can achieve with medications.

I want you to understand that "having very few side effects" does not mean that medications are completely safe over the long term.

I want you to know that medications shown to have statistically significant benefits may not be relevant for your individual situation.

Last, I want you to realize that all doctors and healthcare providers have a bias in the way they practice medicine, me included.

Most commonly, physician bias falls into one of two categories; "less is more," or "more is better."

When it comes to prescriptions, I'm firmly in the "less is more" camp. For instance, I believe that lifestyle interventions should always be the first step, not a prescription. I believe statistics don't tell the whole story. I believe general medication guidelines have little value when considering the individual in front of me. These are my biases.

Other doctors believe just the opposite. It doesn't make one approach right and one wrong. However, if a provider's particular bias doesn't agree with your personal wishes and beliefs, you should feel empowered to question their recommendations and receive an acceptable explanation. That is how you become your own health advocate.

We have numerous opportunities to improve our health with purposeful lifestyle interventions. Numerous opportunities to avoid symptom-masking prescriptions. Numerous opportunities to re-examine our health and our healthcare.

I'll highlight some of the most common examples below.

STATINS

Statins are miracle drugs and should be added to the water supply.

Statins are poison and should never cross your lips!

If you read popular social media posts, you've likely seen both these claims.

How can a single drug be so polarizing?

As a cardiologist, statins are one of the most controversial topics I encounter on a daily basis. They are a prime example of why we need to re-examine our health care and understand the difference between *statistically* significant findings and clinically significant findings. The difference between general guidelines and health care designed for us as an individual.

If a drug shows one half of one percent benefit over five years, that result could very well be statistically significant.

But does it matter for you? If you were considering open heart surgery with significant risk and lengthy recovery time, no way would that tiny benefit be worth it! If you were thinking about eating fish two more times per week, then it might be worth it.

The statistics have to be considered in the context of what the therapy entails—for example, the risk of side effects or what's involved in recovery.

Statins also show us yet again that easy prescriptions are no substitute for actually making purposeful lifestyle changes.

The 2013 American College of Cardiology and American Heart Association cholesterol treatment guidelines dramatically altered mainstream medicine's use of statins. These new recommendations dramatically increased the number of people *without cardiovascular disease* who are eligible for statins, now estimated at 45 million Americans.

Does that mean statins are wonder drugs that we should all take? Definitely not.

It *does* mean that studies support their potential benefit for certain groups of people.

My challenge as a cardiologist is to adequately explain the risks and benefits of statins to patients, to define the degree of potential benefits, and to apply the latest science to the individual person I'm working with.

That's not always easy.

Statins are a billion-dollar-industry supported by hundreds of studies, most of them funded by pharmaceutical companies and designed ahead of time to show maximal benefit. Yet plenty of evidence questioning their benefit and highlighting their potential side effects also exists.

I want to be clear: I use statins without hesitation with many of my patients. My priority, however, is always to determine whether the risk-benefit balance is in the patient's favor before prescribing statins.

I feel medicine as an institution tends to over-emphasize the potential benefits of statins, under-emphasize the potential risks, and completely ignore the alternatives. My goal is to reverse that approach by strongly emphasizing the alternatives, and provide a fair and thorough assessment of the potential benefits and risks.

Cholesterol—not the real enemy

Health, not cholesterol levels, is our primary objective. In reality, high cholesterol has never hurt anyone. What hurts people? Heart attacks and strokes. *Those* are what we want to prevent.

True, elevated cholesterol has been shown to be one of many risk factors associated with cardiovascular disease, but it is clearly an imperfect measurement that does not reliably predict illness or death. It is, however, the easiest to treat with medication and therefore gets the most attention.

In reality, cholesterol is vitally important to our brain function, hormone production, and the integrity of our cell membranes. Without cholesterol in our bodies, there would be no life.

Multiple studies—not all, but more than just a few—have suggested that individuals over age 75

YOUR BEST HEALTH EVER!

are more likely to die if they have *low* cholesterol than if they have high cholesterol, so there is clearly more to the story than simply declaring that cholesterol is evil and must be eliminated.

After all, smoking is likely the most detrimental activity for your health and risk for heart disease. Yet smoking does not increase your "bad" LDL cholesterol concentration. Instead, other factors such as inflammation and oxidation are potentially more important than cholesterol.

Moreover, more than 50% of people with heart attacks have "normal" cholesterol levels and people taking statins still have heart attacks.

In some of the best statin trials, such as the PROVE-IT trial, twenty percent of those taking statins had a heart attack within only two years.

Clearly, statins are not completely protective and cholesterol is not the whole story.

Despite this, I have seen countless patients start a statin who then feel that they've been "treated" and no longer need to pay attention to other heart risk factors. I'm not suggesting they were ever told that they didn't need to worry about nutrition, inactivity or smoking. I'm certain they were not. Yet it is a powerful natural feeling that is difficult to overcome.

In fact, studies have shown that after starting a statin people exercise less, eat more, and gain more weight.

If you decide to take a statin, it's crucial to manage your expectations. Statins are not miracle drugs. They do not "cure" you. They do not single-handedly eliminate your risk of cardiovascular disease. Your LDL may look better on paper, but that is far from the whole picture,

Statins are one very small piece of the puzzle that is your health.

The science

The scientific literature generally shows that statins provide approximately a 30% reduction in heart attacks in high-risk patients, defined as those who have had heart attacks before. Remember, however, that a 30% reduction is the *relative* risk reduction, and not the absolute risk reduction.

In reality, these studies show a 2-3% absolute reduction in heart attacks over a five-year period. There is an even smaller reduction of the risk of death in men, and there is no consistent death benefit seen in women.

That doesn't sound as impressive, does it? It may still be worth it for very high risk people to take a statin, but again, statins are a small piece of the puzzle. They need to be combined with lifestyle interventions as part of a comprehensive treatment plan.

Moreover, those numbers are for high-risk patients (secondary prevention) where we would expect to see the greatest benefit. In people who have not had previous heart attacks (called primary prevention in the medical literature), the benefits are only a 0.5%-1.6% reduction in heart attacks over two to five years. It's statistically significant, but far from earth shattering. And there is no benefit on risk of death.

More importantly, you should consider whether this result is clinically significant for *you*.

If you've already had a heart attack, lowering your risk of another heart attack by 2-3% may be a good enough reason for you to start a statin, even with the risk of potential side effects.

However, if you've never had a heart attack and your risk is not as high, is it still worth it? That's for you to decide, and you deserve to have all the relevant information before you make the decision.

For instance, if you've never had a heart attack before, taking statins for five years does nothing to reduce your risk of death. You need to treat anywhere between 60 and 140 patients for 5 years to prevent one heart attack. That means possibly 99% of the people treated will not see a clinical benefit. You won't see that on the TV commercials.

Will statins make you feel better, more energetic, or stronger? Quite the opposite. Statins have been shown to decrease exercise activity, worsen sleep patterns, and increase daily aches and pains.

You have to ask yourself why you'd start taking a drug if it didn't reduce your risk of death and didn't make you feel better.

One argument is that statins are "the best we have" for reducing cardiovascular risk. If you're talking about the best available drug choice, manufactured in a factory, that may be true. But if you consider the wealth of lifestyle choices available to us on a daily basis, I would argue that statins are far from "the best we have to offer."

Cholesterol...or inflammation?

If cholesterol isn't the real enemy, what is? We must have some enemy to blame, right? It turns out inflammation might fit that role.

The widely-known JUPITER trial studied the role of statins in primary prevention—preventing heart attacks in people who had never had one. This trial specifically looked at people with elevated hs-CRP, a lab marker of inflammation, and relatively normal or minimally elevated LDL cholesterol levels. Researchers treated study participants with either the statin rosuvastatin or a placebo.

They stopped the trial after only two years because they reached a statistically significant finding that statins reduced cardiovascular events by 0.6% over the two-year period. That means you need to treat 166 people for two years to prevent one cardiovascular event. That's not terribly impressive—yet this finding was publicized as a blockbuster breakthrough.

Again, the important question is whether this statistically significant difference is clinically significant. And are there other potential treatments that are equally as effective or even more effective?

It turns out that in addition to reducing cholesterol, statins also reduce inflammation. In fact, analysis of the study's data suggests that the beneficial effect of statins was *only seen* in those who had a reduction in their hs-CRP inflammation marker. Those who lowered their LDL, but not their hs-CRP, did not seem to benefit.

This finding suggests that lower inflammation, not lower LDL, may have been the primary reason for reduced heart attack risk.

Indeed, chronic inflammation appears to be a much more likely cause of cardiovascular complications than LDL levels in isolation.

It's becoming more evident that not all plaques—deposits in arteries—are the same. And neither are all LDL particles. Oxidized and inflamed plaques appear to be more likely to cause heart attacks compared to less inflamed plaques. The same holds true for oxidized and inflamed LDL particles.

Therefore, other methods of reducing plaque and lipid inflammation should be equally as beneficial for reducing heart attacks as would statins. After all, smoking cessation, regular exercise, stress reduction and proper nutrition have all been shown to reduce inflammation **and** to reduce heart attacks. It certainly seems like we're on to something there!

What will statins do for you?

One very important point I stress with my clients is that we do not know what effect statins have on people who follow proper lifestyle choices. Almost all the major statin studies were done with individuals who eat a low-fat/high-carbohydrate high-sugar diet, and pay little attention to lifestyle interventions.

Well, guess what? Both the standard American diet, as well as the low-fat high-carb diet, have been shown to increase inflammation and promote oxidation. That's exactly what we're trying to prevent! It should be no surprise, therefore, that statins would show a benefit in that setting.

The next question is obvious. What if you purposefully minimized your body's inflammation with healthy eating, stress reduction, regular exercise and restorative sleep? I believe statins would probably have minimal, if any, benefit under those improved lifestyle circumstances.

Unfortunately, since that finding wouldn't be in the best interest of drug companies, we're unlikely to ever see that study get adequate funding to be done properly. That's why we need individual voices screaming this from the rooftops.

We don't need drugs to accomplish what we can do better with lifestyle!!!

In fact, a 2016 study in the New England Journal of Medicine showed that lifestyle interventions can reduce the risk of heart disease in those at highest genetic risk by almost 50%. And guess what? These benefits were accomplished with minimal if any change in the LDL.

Remember the PREDIMED study that showed the Mediterranean diet reduces cardiovascular events? It also showed a significant benefit with no meaningful reduction in LDL.

I'll say it again. We don't need drugs to accomplish what we can do better with lifestyle!!!

Adverse effects of statins

Why do some say statins are poison and should be avoided at all costs? While that is likely an

YOUR BEST HEALTH EVER!

overstatement, like most drugs, statins do have significant potential side effects.

Significant statin-induced muscle aches or weakness have been reported in at least 10% of users. Anecdotal "real world" reports are as high as 50% in some settings, especially in active individuals.

In fact, statin users tend to decrease their exercise after starting the medication. That's right: the drug most often prescribed to reduce cardiovascular risk can cause patients to exercise less! Sounds counterproductive to me.

In very rare cases the muscle damage may be life-threatening, although fortunately the incidence dropped dramatically after an older statin, Baycol, was removed from the market in 2001.

In most cases, the muscle aches are a nuisance that may limit your physical activity. Biopsy studies, however, do suggest muscle cell damage even in the absence of abnormal lab results. More research is likely forthcoming on this topic.

Rarely, statins cause liver dysfunction. However, it's easy to monitor for this side effect and liver function returns to normal when the drug is stopped.

Of greatest concern to most of my clients, however, are the risks for diabetes and dementia.

The risk of statin-associated Type 2 diabetes is fortunately not high. Studies showed that treating between 166 individuals and 250 individuals with a statin for two years would result in one new case of diabetes. But for a low-risk individual, this could be significantly greater than the potential benefit of the drug.

In addition, it concerns me that the "long-term" studies done on statins have only lasted 5-6 years.

That's not very reassuring at a time when we're often starting 30- and 40-year-olds on statins.

They could be on them for 40+ years!

If the increase in the risk of diabetes is significant, the 10- and 20-year data may look much different, as more people suffer the complications from their accelerated diabetes.

As you read earlier, cholesterol is essential for proper neurological function. It should be no surprise, therefore, that reducing it puts our brains at risk for dementia.

Since statins are used most often in an aging population, and some degree of memory loss happens naturally as we age, it is difficult to know exactly how many people suffer cognitive decline from statins.

It's becoming more clear, however, that it is a significant concern and will likely increase in the future as our population continues to age and the use of statins continues to increase.

So are statins poison that should be avoided at all costs? Of course not.

Are they perfect drugs? Most definitely not.

They are somewhere in between, and the potential benefits need to be weighed against an honest assessment of the potential risks.

What if a statin is recommended?

Given all this information, what can you do if your physician recommends you start a statin based on your calculated risk?

The first step is to recognize that taking a statin is not a black-and-white issue. It requires a meticulous patient-by-patient analysis of the benefits, risks and alternatives to statins.

Some individuals value the potential benefits from statins no matter how small they may be, while others are more concerned with potential side effects, no matter how small they may be.

The only certainty is that there are no absolute criteria for taking a statin. Even the newest guidelines emphasize that those at risk should start the *discussion* about taking a statin. They do not say that you should definitively take one. It is a subjective decision that you should make based on your individual interpretation of objective data in partnership with your doctor.

Before prescribing, I would always ask "What else can be done to enhance the evaluation of your individual risk for heart disease?"

The guidelines mention that in addition to the calculated risk, physicians may want to consider:

- ⊙ The person's family history of premature heart disease
- ⊙ The high-sensitivity CRP (hs-CRP) inflammation blood test
- ⊙ The ankle-brachial (ABI) test for peripheral vascular disease

⊙   An elevated coronary calcium score
    that is above 300 or above the 75th
    percentile for age

Amazingly, the recommendation is to use these
tests only for deciding in favor of statins. The
guidelines don't mention, for example, using a
calcium score of zero to eliminate the need for
statin therapy. They don't mention using a normal
ABI and a normal hs-CRP as evidence that your risk
is lower, and you therefore don't need statins.

Why not? Likely because the guideline authors
have a bias towards initiating statin therapy—the
"more is better" approach. Believing that more
medicine is always better is a very common bias
in medicine that comes from the desire to help.
Unfortunately, it's not always best for your health.

I take the opposite approach. What if our bias is
against starting a statin?

A trial published in the Journal of the American
College of Cardiology looked at that exact question.
They found that about 50% of the people aged 45-75
who met other criteria for starting a statin also had
a calcium score of 0.

Factoring this calcium score into their risk analysis
reclassifies them into a lower-risk category that no
longer meets the threshold for statin therapy.

That's a lot of statin prescriptions that could be
avoided, thus reducing the cost and risk to the
patient.

We need to re-examine how we approach risk
assessment. We should look for reasons to promote
lifestyle and not promote drugs. That's not what
the pharmaceutical industry wants. That is what I

want, and that is what you should want, for your health and for your safety, now and for a lifetime.

Don't forget about HDL

HDL cholesterol was once considered the holy grail for medical interventions. If low HDL was a risk factor for developing heart disease, then raising it must be protective, right? The search for the miracle drug began.

Drug companies invested millions of dollars developing a class of drugs called "CETP inhibitors," which raise HDL and lower LDL. It seemed like a simple solution. The trials, however, have consistently shown no cardiovascular benefits from these drugs despite their "improvement" in HDL and LDL. In fact, some trials showed a potential harm from their use with an increased risk of death!

Even the vitamin niacin, which increases HDL, has yet to show any significant reduction in cardiovascular events.

How could this be?

Some would argue that HDL must not be that important. In fact, a 2016 publication questioned the benefits of HDL, but likely missed the most important point. Improving your lab values with drugs is not the same as making lifestyle changes which improve your health. It's not the HDL that is the goal. It is the activities, the nutritional choices, and the lifestyle we lead that is the goal. The HDL just happens to follow those healthy choices.

Regular exercise, including resistance training, can naturally raise HDL. In addition, a high-fat nutrient-dense diet can naturally raise HDL. As it turns out, these interventions do reduce your risk of cardiovascular disease.

Once again, we are unlikely to see that recommendation in a TV commercial. Instead of promoting expensive drugs that don't work well and in some cases even harm you, we need to promote proven lifestyle changes whose only side effects are more energy, feeling better, and being healthier!

Consider advanced lipid testing

All LDL and HDL are not created equal.

This is why the familiar cholesterol test that checks your LDL, HDL and triglyceride (TG) concentration only scratches the surface of what's important to know about your cholesterol profile.

Some types of LDL may be more dangerous, or atherogenic, than others. For instance, the degree of oxidation and inflammation of LDL particles increases the risk of cardiovascular events.

There's also a difference between large and small LDL particles, and a difference between the concentration of LDL and the absolute number of LDL particles in your blood. For instance, small LDL particles may be a better predictor for cardiovascular disease than the total amount of cholesterol in your blood.

A higher LDL concentration of larger, less dangerous LDL particles is less concerning than the lower concentration of small, more dangerous particles commonly seen in those with diabetes, metabolic syndrome, and insulin resistance.

Only advanced lipid testing can measure these elements.

To be fair, the evidence is not uniformly in favor of advanced lipid testing. The American College of Cardiology and the American Heart Association state that the evidence does not support the added expense of routine advanced lipid testing for the general population. Many insurance carriers, therefore, will not pay for these tests and your doctor may not recommend advanced lipid testing. That doesn't make him or her wrong. In fact, they'd simply be following the guidelines—guidelines that were developed with the bias that more statin use is a good thing.

As you now know, that is by no means the only valid perspective.

I find advanced lipid testing very useful for showing people that they may not benefit from statins.

Here's a scenario that happens frequently in my practice. A 50-year old executive without heart disease hears from his doctor that, based on his risk calculation, he should start a statin. He sees me for a second opinion and I order advanced lipid tests.

If I find that his LDL particle number is low, and the LDL are larger and less atherogenic, and their oxidation and inflammation are low, right away I can see he's at lower risk than initially thought.

Combine that with a low coronary calcium score and attention to meaningful lifestyle changes, and suddenly a statin is no longer even on our radar screen.

In addition, advanced lipid testing also helps me understand how you respond to various interventions.

For instance, your LDL may not change much when you start exercising and improving your nutritional choices. Traditionally, we'd label that a "failure of lifestyle changes." We might even suspect that you were fibbing about your exercise routine or your food choices.

But what if, after you started exercising and eating better, your HDL went up, your LDL particle number went down, your LDL particles were no longer small and dense, and your LDL was now much less oxidized and inflamed—all despite no change in your overall LDL concentration?

That is the *exact* response I hope to see as a result of purposeful lifestyle changes. I would call that a tremendous success and a fantastic response!

Standard lipid testing, however, will miss all those beneficial changes.

I understand why insurance carriers may not pay for these tests, but on a patient-by-patient basis I frequently find that the more detailed information is well worth the extra cost for patients committed to reducing their heart disease risk.

Check your coronary calcium score

As mentioned above, a coronary calcium score is an invaluable tool for cardiac risk assessment. Those with a calcium score of zero have less than 1% risk of a cardiac event over 5-years. A zero score can also alter the risk calculation in 50% of individuals so that they no longer "qualify" for a statin.

To be fair, calcium scores are not perfect tests. They have radiation, a low dose of less than half the amount you get on a cross-country flight. They are usually not covered by insurance; the cost is about $100. They may show incidental findings that require future follow-up, like benign findings in the lung or liver.

Despite these potential downsides, they can be a welcome addition to improve the assessment of your cardiac risk.

We can do better than a drug!

The guidelines don't know what to do with you! Don't accept a statin prescription without further defining your risk. In the end, it may be appropriate for you to start a statin. But don't decide based on the knee-jerk reaction that more medicine is always better.

If you're practicing mindfulness techniques, getting adequate restorative sleep, exercising regularly, and following a nutrient-dense high quality veggie-based diet, you've likely already done most (if not all) of the statin's work.

You can do better than a drug!

PROTON PUMP INHIBITORS

Gastroesophageal reflux disease (GERD) is a chronic digestive disorder that occurs when stomach acid flows backwards—"refluxes"— into your esophagus, the tube that leads to your stomach.

Treating GERD is a $10 billion industry with fifteen million Americans currently take proton pump inhibitor (PPI) drugs. PPIs work by reducing the amount of acid that your stomach produces, thus preventing potential damage to the esophagus and reducing the reflux-related pain.

Healthcare providers have historically considered PPIs to be safe. In reality, that may not be completely true. In fact, PPIs are a prime example of a clinical band-aid that masks the symptoms without addressing the underlying cause of the problem.

Originally, PPIs were recommended for only 6 – 8 weeks of use. Their main purpose was to heal the damage to the esophagus caused by reflux, while doctor and patient worked together to find and eliminate the underlying cause of the reflux.

Over time, however, doctors and patients began relying on PPIs as long-term treatment for GERD, abandoning efforts to resolve the underlying causes. Even worse, because PPIs eliminated heartburn symptoms, many people felt that they now had a license to eat whatever they wanted— which only worsened the underlying causes of their heartburn.

Unanticipated consequences

Our bodies need stomach acid to digest food, activate digestive enzymes in our small intestine and to help absorb vitamins and nutrients. Reducing stomach acid, therefore, is not natural and is not harmless.

In fact, reducing stomach acid has been linked to a higher risk of infections like pneumonia and the potentially deadly intestinal infection clostridium difficile as well as vitamin deficiencies, dementia and kidney disease.

YOUR BEST HEALTH EVER!

A study in Germany followed over 73,000 people 75 years old or older and found that those who took PPIs had a 44% increased risk of dementia compared with those who were not taking PPIs. Another, earlier, study showed increased risk of kidney disease in PPI users compared to non-users.

As we mentioned previously, an observational study that shows an association between two elements does not prove that one caused the other. These two studies did not *prove* that PPIs cause dementia or kidney disease. It's certainly possible, but not proven.

It's also plausible that there is something about the heartburn itself, rather than the medication, that causes dementia or kidney disease. Or maybe it's because people with heartburn tend to be heavier, eat worse diets, exercise less, smoke more, or have a myriad of other unhealthy habits that increase the risk for chronic diseases.

All we know for sure is that there is something about people who have GERD and take PPIs that places them at higher risk for these conditions.

The overall solution, therefore, should be to institute lifestyle changes to eliminate the underlying cause of GERD. That, in turn, lets you eliminate the need for PPIs in the first place. Now, it no longer matters whether the problem was GERD or PPIs. You've gotten rid of both, thus removing all the potential negative long-term health effects!

Solving the underlying problem

The solution for GERD is to keep the acid in the stomach, where it belongs, and to prevent it from going into the esophagus, where it does not belong.

In some people, an anatomical or physical problem causes GERD, and requires aggressive medical or surgical care. For example, a severe hiatal hernia, where part of the stomach slips into the chest, may require surgery. Rare conditions where the stomach aggressively overproduces acid will require medication.

For most of us, however, seven purposeful lifestyle adjustments will reduce acid reflux into the esophagus without reducing the necessary acid within the stomach.

⊙ Do not eat within two hours of going to bed

If we eat shortly before we lie down, our full stomach is more likely to reflux.

Gravity is your friend when it comes to keeping the acid in your stomach, where it belongs. In addition, we often eat more sugary or processed foods late at night. Remember the "after 7 p.m." eating dilemma I referenced earlier? These poor nutritional choices can also lead to more reflux.

⊙ Eat smaller meals

Acid is less likely to reflux back into your esophagus when your stomach is less full and distended. Eat to relieve hunger, not to feel full.

⊙ Avoid alcohol, caffeine, fried foods, mint and chocolate

These specific foods can relax the lower esophageal sphincter (LES). The job of the LES is to prevent stomach acid from entering the esophagus. Relaxing it, therefore, allows reflux to occur.

⊙ Stop smoking

Cigarette smoke greatly increases the risk of reflux. But to be honest, if you're still smoking, reflux is the least of your health concerns.

⊙ Maintain an ideal body weight

It's especially important to reduce abdominal fat and visceral fat around your internal organs as these are greatly associated with reflux.

⊙ Treat H. pylori infections

This is a common stomach infection that's easily treated with a two-week course of antibiotics. If you are having trouble with chronic GERD, ask your physician about testing for H. Pylori infection.

⊙ Address stress

You know what else increases GERD? Getting married. Getting divorced. Getting fired. Starting a new job. Final exams. And more.

What do all these have in common? STRESS!

Fortunately, practicing the stress management and relaxation techniques in Chapter 6 can help reduce GERD symptoms.

In addition, magnesium supplements offer a simple treatment with few serious side effects. Magnesium has been shown to both improve our bodies' reaction to stress and the symptoms of GERD. Therefore, in addition to a consistent mindful practice, I recommend magnesium supplements to most of my clients with increased stress, GERD, or both.

Food, food, food

When GERD doesn't respond to purposeful lifestyle changes, the most likely cause is actual food sensitivities. When our bodies cannot efficiently digest our food, it sits in our stomach longer, causing more stomach acid secretion, and increasing the risk of reflux.

Food intolerances are different for everyone, but the two most common are gluten and dairy. Other common intolerances are soy and legumes.

The best way to identify the culprit is to start by eliminating these items from your diet. Then, slowly re-introduce specific classes of food and assess whether your GERD improves or worsens. While logistically challenging, the elimination diet is the best way to find the true cause of GERD.

....

Check Yourself for Food Sensitivities

If your GERD has not responded to lifestyle changes, start an elimination diet.

Get rid of all gluten, dairy, soy and legumes.

Did your GERD improve? If so, slowly add back one item at a time until you find the ones that make it worse. You will have your culprit and know what to avoid. Knowledge is power.

....

If it doesn't improve, then you likely need a more detailed evaluation with an experienced nutritionist or functional medicine provider. They may want to test for conditions such as small intestine bacterial overgrowth or "leaky gut" syndrome. Both of these conditions are on the forefront of research into potential causes of GERD. Much of this investigation is taking shape outside of mainstream medicine. That doesn't make it wrong—it just means that it may take longer to gain popular acceptance.

Conclusion

Looking back at all these contributors to GERD, I can see why some doctors and patients prefer to start a PPI and get rid of the symptoms right away. Quick relief of symptoms is hard to turn down—even when it leaves your real health issue untreated and exposes you to new health risks.

And that's why doing the challenging work of becoming a lifestyle and nutrition detective is so important. Masking the symptoms doesn't improve your health. It just gives you a false sense of security.

Don't trade one problem—heartburn symptoms— for another problem—long-term medications and their side effects. You deserve to have someone spend the time to help you get to your GERD's root cause and *eliminate* it.

OTHER EXAMPLES

Opportunities to re-examine your healthcare abound, as these brief examples illustrate:

Type 2 diabetes

Most diabetes medications increase your insulin levels. However, insulin is a fat storage hormone. You therefore gain fat weight on these medications, which can worsen your diabetes and require higher doses of medication.

Regular exercise, good sleep patterns, and proper nutrition can improve your body's ability to use glucose and require less insulin, thus treating your diabetes without the side effects of medications. In fact, studies have shown that a lower carbohydrate diet can improve diabetes control and lower the need for medication.

Again, we see that lifestyle changes can do just as well as most medicines. The bonus is that a healthy lifestyle has *beneficial* side effects. It also treats your heart disease, your blood pressure and more. Diabetes drugs can't boast those same benefits!

Depression

It's estimated that 19 million Americans, approximately 9% of the population, suffer from depression in any given year. Depression most commonly comes from an imbalance of chemicals deep within our brain. The usual treatment, therefore, is to prescribe drugs to reset those chemicals.

You may be surprised to hear that lifestyle interventions are as effective as medications at treating the symptoms of mild and moderate depression.

For instance, plant-based, Mediterranean-style eating can significantly improve depression symptoms, whereas high-carbohydrate and high-sugar meals tend to worsen them.

Think about it. If you have a high-carb/high-sugar meal, chances are you're not very satisfied an hour after the meal. You'll likely be hungry again, and craving more carbs.

What will those cravings do to your mood? You guessed it. Irritable, grumpy and depressed. On the other hand, plant-based, whole food, Mediterranean-based meals full of healthy fats reduce your cravings, keep you full, and avoid the irritable mood swings. That's likely not the only way nutrition benefits depression symptoms, but it certainly helps!

Regular exercise is also as effective as prescription medications for the control of mild to moderate depression.

Once again, however, we find it's often quicker and easier to prescribe an antidepressant pill—despite a laundry list of side effects including sexual dysfunction, drowsiness, reports of emotional "numbness" and many others. Just thinking about those side effects depresses me!

We don't have to give in to the quick fix. Science supports our decision to take charge of our own treatment with purposeful lifestyle interventions.

Once again, we can do better than prescription drugs!

Low back pain

Studies consistently show no significant improvement in low back pain symptoms when surgical intervention is compared to physical therapy and lifestyle interventions.

Yet there is a pervasive feeling in medicine that if we aren't "doing something," we aren't doing everything we can to help you. Therefore, the bias is towards surgery because it's more active, more immediate, and gives everyone the sense that we're doing "all that we can."

I maintain that purposeful lifestyle changes and physical therapy is doing more. Those are the interventions that help you heal and keep you healthy in the long run.

CONCLUSION

Sometimes medications are necessary and can be lifesaving. More often, they're better replaced with purposeful lifestyle changes. Ask your medical provider if they're willing to work with you on lifestyle as the primary treatment option.

When you treat yourself with purposeful lifestyle interventions, you can often meet or beat the benefits of medications, and you have the added psychological benefit of knowing that *you* are in charge of your health.

Not a pill. Not a doctor. You.

That's priceless.

THE PLAN: RE-EXAMINE YOUR HEALTHCARE

Week 1

- ⊙ Know your baseline blood tests. At a minimum, get a standard lipid panel, hs-CRP test, fasting glucose and insulin levels, and Vitamin D level.

⊙ Even better, discuss with your doctor the option of getting advanced lipid testing

⊙ Measure your baseline weight, BMI, waist circumference, and body fat percentage.

⊙ Carefully review your medications with your physician. Inform him or her that you intend to implement purposeful lifestyle changes to safely decrease your dependence on them.

Week 2

⊙ Consider whether supplements are needed, based on your lab values and nutritional habits. See Resources for an in-depth discussion of supplements.

Week 3

⊙ Investigate local functional medicine practitioners or other practitioners who take a whole-patient approach and value lifestyle interventions. If you find you're hitting too many roadblocks, you may want to arrange a consultation.

Week 4

⊙ Recheck your labs and reassess your need for prescription medications. Do you really need to treat your cholesterol, blood pressure, diabetes, heartburn, etc., with drugs? Or have lifestyle changes already shown that you could potentially fix the underlying problems?

⊙ Re-measure your weight, BMI and body fat percentage. You're not setting goals. You're simply updating your earlier baseline to track early progress.

———

For journal citations and more insight into the PROVE-IT and JUPITER studies of statins and heart attack risk, studies of GERD, diabetes and depression, and other research from this chapter, visit the Book Resources Blog at DrBretScher.com.

———

Conclusion

There you have it. The surprisingly simple roadmap to your best health ever.

Everything in this book is doable. You can take charge of your health. And you can start now.

Your success starts with your mindset. Believe that you can change and believe that you can improve. Break the negative cycle that expects disappointment, and move yourself into the space where you implement what you've learned.

You won't be perfect, and you shouldn't expect to be perfect. The journey is lifelong. Commit to doing it better, and getting healthier, every day. You'll be amazed by the improvements you can make, and delighted at how much better you can feel.

Some of the information I've covered was probably new to you, and some of it was probably a reminder of things you already knew. Find ways to embrace what you've learned, prioritize it, and incorporate it into your life.

That sounds easier than it is, which is why it's crucial to implement numerous daily reminders. We need to remind ourselves why we want to be healthy, what we hope to achieve, and how we plan to create the habits to get us there and keep us there.

Once you are in the right space to succeed, then you can focus on your nutrition, your physical activity, your stress management and sleep, and you can build your community of support and guidance.

You'll have all the tools in place to allow you to live the life you want.

A life free of medication dependency.

A life where your health is manifest in all your daily habits.

A life where you achieve your best health ever!

Resources

The 12-Week Roadmap to Natural Health

THE PLAN: MODIFY YOUR MINDSET

Week 1

⊙ Define your goals, write them down and sign the paper. Take time to visualize what it looks like to accomplish those goals. Remember to visualize the habits that coincide with achieving those goals, too. Start asking your positively framed "What if" questions.

Week 2

⊙ Develop a personal statement that resonates with you and helps establish your path to healthy habits. Say this statement aloud when you wake up every day to help set your intention for the day. Along the same lines, search for both your short-term and long-term purpose.

Week 3

⊙ Add a simple daily action to remind you of your goals and your purpose. Perform this action every day and celebrate it. It doesn't count if you don't celebrate it!

Week 4

⊙ Start an accountability calendar. Review it on a weekly basis to celebrate your successes and spot opportunities for improvement.

THE PLAN: NOURISH YOUR BODY

Week 1

⊙ Become more mindful with everything you eat. Ask yourself, what nutrition does it provide? Does it help you feel full and feel energized? Do you enjoy it? Does it help you or hurt you?

⊙ Practice mindful techniques when you eat. Start each meal with three mindful breaths, and focus on your food as you eat. Use this to help you assess your fullness, so you stop eating when you're no longer hungry.

Week 2

⊙ Make this a week of eating 100% real food. You need to see how good you can feel with a 100% real food diet.

⊙ Everything you eat should be from the earth or an animal, not a factory.

Focus on real food, real veggies and real proteins/fats.

⊙ Detox your kitchen. Focus on the quality of what surrounds you. Control your environment by eliminating all non-real food, sweets, liquid calories, added sugars, and processed food.

⊙ It's just for a week. You can do it!

Week 3

⊙ Experiment with intermittent fasting one or two days per week. The easiest way is to stop eating at 6 or 7 p.m. Don't eat again until noon the next day.

⊙ Learn that you can control your hunger physically and psychologically.

⊙ Use a nutrient tracker like My Fitness Pal to track calories, protein, fat and carbohydrates. Don't worry about hitting targets or certain percentages. This is for your information only.

Week 4

⊙ Research potential restaurants where you can comfortably eat out.

⊙ Pick two or three "go to" restaurants and one or two menu items that work for your real food eating plan.

⊙ Repeat your week of 100% real food and see how much easier it is a second time.

THE PLAN: MOVE WITH PURPOSE

Here's the core principle behind this plan: when you exercise with purpose and intensity three days each week, and use your activity tracker to make sure you're moving more the rest of the week, you don't need formal exercise every single day to achieve better health and lower your risk of chronic diseases.

Week 1

⊙ Increase your daily activity: park farther away, take the stairs, walk every 30 minutes at work, start a gardening project, etc.

⊙ Get an activity tracker and determine your baseline activity level.

Week 2

⊙ Start exercising daily for at least 15 minutes. That's it. Just 15 minutes. Walk when you get up, before dinner, at lunch. Just 15 minutes.

⊙ Pay attention to how your daily exercise changes your activity monitor data

⊙ Begin daily functional alignment exercises.

Week 3

⊙ Set your goal on your activity monitor. Shoot for at least 8,000-12,000 steps per day, keeping in mind that more is better. Adjust your goal according to your baseline activity level.

- ⊙ Exercise 30 minutes three days per week.

- ⊙ Continue daily posture exercises.

Week 4

- ⊙ Pick two of your exercise days and substitute high-intensity interval training and strength training on those days.

- ⊙ Consider starting off with a trainer or a fitness program

- ⊙ Make sure you're still hitting your activity monitor goals at least five days per week. If not, formulate a specific plan for achieving that goal.

THE PLAN: MANAGE YOUR STRESS & SLEEP

Week 1

- ⊙ Practice becoming mindful during your daily activities. Practice being in the present.

- ⊙ Pay attention to the stressors in your daily life and notice how you respond to stress. Take note. Do you clench your teeth or your fists? Do you feel an uneasy sensation in your stomach?

- ⊙ Start to breathe first, before you respond, and see how it changes your physical response to the stressor.

Week 2

- ⊙ Create your welcoming and peaceful sleep retreat.

- ⊙ Create pleasing sensations with pictures, smells or sounds.

- ⊙ Keep your room cool and completely dark.

- ⊙ Remove activities from the bedroom.

- ⊙ Eliminate screen time one-hour before bedtime.

- ⊙ Set a consistent sleep schedule.

- ⊙ Repeat your positive statement that your bedroom is your peaceful sleep retreat.

Week 3

- ⊙ Start sitting for a five-minute meditation session.

- ⊙ Make this a consistent schedule so that you sit at the same time every day. You can do it when you wake up, when you're about to go to sleep, during your lunch break, or anytime that's quiet.

- ⊙ Don't wait for a crazy moment when you need to calm yourself down. Meditation is preventive and mind-forming, not crisis management. Remember, it is not about doing it right or wrong. The process is the goal.

Week 4

- ⊙ Increase your meditation sessions to 10 minutes and include mindful practices in your daily activities.

- ⊙ Focus on your breathing during work, during your walks, and especially during times of stress or struggle.

- ⊙ Focus on being present and breathing.

THE PLAN: BUILD YOUR SUPPORT COMMUNITY

Week 1

- ⊙ Talk about your goals with your friends and loved ones.

- ⊙ Gauge their responses. Are they supportive, or dubious? Constructive, or critical?

- ⊙ Use this feedback to help you decide who to include in your community, and enroll at least two people the first week

Week 2

- ⊙ Expand your community to your workplace and your local neighborhood

- ⊙ Communicate your goals with your healthcare providers and explore what support they may provide.

Week 3

- ⊙ Explore online communities, through activity trackers, social media sites, message forums and elsewhere to expand your reach, increase learning opportunities, and explore new aspects of your health journey.

Week 4

⊙ Celebrate as a community. Have a formal celebration event and define the successes you are choosing to celebrate. Don't forget, you are celebrating your support community as much as they are celebrating your successes.

THE PLAN: RE-EXAMINE YOUR HEALTHCARE

Week 1

⊙ Know your baseline blood tests. At a minimum, get a standard lipid panel, hs-CRP test, fasting glucose and insulin levels, and Vitamin D level.

⊙ Even better, discuss with your doctor the option of getting advanced lipid testing

⊙ Measure your baseline weight, BMI, waist circumference, and body fat percentage.

⊙ Carefully review your medications with your physician. Inform him or her that you intend to implement purposeful lifestyle changes to safely decrease your dependence on them.

Week 2

⊙ Consider whether supplements are needed, based on your lab values and nutritional habits. See Resources for an in-depth discussion of supplements.

Week 3

⊙ Investigate local functional medicine practitioners or other practitioners who take a whole-patient approach and value lifestyle interventions. If you find you're hitting too many roadblocks, you may want to arrange a consultation.

Week 4

⊙ Recheck your labs and reassess your need for prescription medications. Do you really need to treat your cholesterol, blood pressure, diabetes, heartburn, etc., with drugs? Or have lifestyle changes already shown that you could potentially fix the underlying problems?

⊙ Re-measure your weight, BMI and body fat percentage. You're not setting goals. You're simply updating your earlier baseline to track early progress.

The Tune-up Checklist

Your four-week program helps you lay the groundwork for a lifetime of success. It introduces the tools, gives you time to become comfortable with them over the course of a week, and then challenges you with a new set of objectives for the following week.

After you complete the first four weeks, I encourage you to go back to the beginning.

Review the steps from each week and spend more time with the ones that proved more difficult.

It may take 8–12 weeks or even longer to complete all the objectives with confidence and mastery.

That's perfectly fine. The key is to ingrain them into who you are so that they become part of your everyday life.

EVERY THREE MONTHS

Take a few minutes and complete the following self-assessment. This process will help you stay on track and anticipate potential pitfalls in time to avoid them.

Mindset

We started your mindset program by writing down your goals and taking ownership by signing them. Every three months, revisit those goals. You may find that your goals have changed. If that's the case, write down your new goals, date them and sign them.

Over time you can notate if you accomplished your goals, if they're ongoing, or if they've changed.

As you did before, continue to visualize achieving your goals, and visualize the steps it takes to get there.

Next, revisit your daily affirmation and your simple action.

Have you maintained these practices? If not, why not?

Make changes to help you maintain the practice over the next three months. Schedule it into your day. Don't leave it to chance that you'll remember to do it.

Fight the fixed mindset and negative feedback loop by looking for opportunities to reaffirm your growth mindset every day. Embrace new challenges and new opportunities for growth.

Nutrition

Every quarter, perform a kitchen clean-out. You'll be surprised at what builds up in three months.

Pick a Sunday, gather your spouse and kids, and go to work. Get rid of the processed, added-sugar, refined-carb foods. Replenish your kitchen so it's full of real, from the earth food.

The clean-out helps you see up close and personal where you've strayed from the Real Food plan. Reaffirm your commitment to eating vegetable based, Mediterranean-style, real foods.

After the clean-out, take time to appreciate your food again. Reignite your mindful eating practice, recognizing the nutrition your food provides, where it came from, and how it was prepared.

Last, grade yourself on your eating-out behaviors. Look back at your most common restaurants and ask yourself if there are better menu choices then the ones you've been gravitating to.

Exercise

People sometimes get bored or frustrated with exercise. Take stock of your weekly exercise routine. Write down what you enjoy and what works, and what you loathe and what doesn't work. Take this opportunity to infuse more excitement in your exercise routine. Make it fun, make it social, keep it up.

If your activity tracker found its way to the bottom of your drawer, dust it off and charge it up. People are frequently surprised to see that their daily steps have trailed off. Use it as a motivator to increase your daily activity.

Remind yourself to get outside and be active!

Walk or bike whenever possible.

Have you started taking the elevator more often? Get back to the stairs.

Are you looking for "rockstar parking?" Go back to parking like you drive a Tesla!

Remind yourself to move your body.

Sleep and stress

It can be a challenge to maintain a consistent meditation and mindfulness practice. If you've maintained your mindfulness practice, celebrate! Rejoice in your commitment and success. If you haven't been able to maintain it, be specific about why not. Pick a specific time each day to restart your practice. Don't leave it up to a last-minute decision. Plan for success.

Reassess your sleep retreat. Is it still an inviting retreat for relaxation and sleep? Has any technology crept its way into your retreat? Change and adapt your sleep retreat to make it as inviting as possible.

Re-examine your healthcare

Continuously re-examine whether the medications you're taking are truly necessary. Make sure your lab work is up to date and that you have regular touchpoints with your healthcare providers.

Remember, your weight is less important than your waist circumference and how your clothes fit. Your weight is also less important than your body fat percentage, your blood sugar and insulin levels, and your amount of inflammation.

ONCE EVERY YEAR

When you reach your one-year anniversary, go back through the entire program, Week 1 through Week 4, to help you reset, regroup and recharge.

Maintain this annual "rinse and repeat" cycle to protect the strong foundation of habits that support your lifetime of health.

The more you reaffirm your commitment, the more a healthy lifestyle becomes who you truly are. That's the path to success.

YOUR TUNE-UP CHECKLIST

Every Three Months

Mindset

- Revisit your mindset goals.
- Update goals that have changed, date them, and sign them.
- Revisit your daily affirmation and your simple action. Update as needed to help you maintain this practice over the next three months.
- Look for daily opportunities to reaffirm your growth mindset with new challenges and opportunities.

Nutrition

- Perform a kitchen clean-out. Take note of what has "crept back in" that isn't real food.
- Reignite your mindful eating practice. Appreciate the nourishment your food provides. Eliminate distracted eating.
- Grade yourself on your eating-out behaviors and look for improvement opportunities.

Exercise

⊙ Take stock of your weekly exercise routine. If you've fallen out of a routine, look for specific reasons, and make a plan to try again.

⊙ If you aren't using your activity tracker regularly, restart this practice.

⊙ Remind yourself to move your body regularly.

Sleep and stress

⊙ Celebrate successes in maintaining your mindfulness practice.

⊙ Commit to restart your practice if you've struggled to maintain it.

⊙ Reassess your sleep retreat and adapt it to make it as inviting as possible.

Build your support community

⊙ Remember to celebrate as a community every three months. Celebrations help re-engage the community and remind everyone about the path you're on.

⊙ Continue to expand your community with new friends you've met.

⊙ Look for opportunities to mentor others within your community.

Re-examine your healthcare

⊙ Re-examine whether the medications you're taking are truly necessary.

⊙ Update your lab work and check in with your healthcare providers.

Every Year

- ⊙ Kick off your anniversary by returning to Week 1

- ⊙ As you progress through each week anew, update your goals for each of the six building blocks

- ⊙ Draw on the experience, insights and learning you've accumulated during the past 12 months.

Troubleshooting Your Plan

Sometimes patients or clients will tell me that "This plan just isn't working for me."

If you feel that this plan isn't working for you, use your growth mindset to focus on the specifics. What didn't work? Be as detailed as possible and write it down. The step of writing it down is very important. It forces you to take ownership of the issue and helps you formulate a plan to overcome it.

Don't settle for vague, general statements like the example above. That causes your mindset to turn toward the negative and isn't very helpful.

EXERCISE OBSTACLES

You're not happy with your exercise progress.

Don't:

- ⊙ Say "The exercise program didn't work for me."

Do write down specific issues, like:

- ⊙ You were not able to get to the gym three days each week

- So you only exercised one day per week
- You always felt tired and sore

That's much more specific—and now you can start to see potential solutions.

Going to the gym may not be the best choice for you. Instead, start with more manageable goals, like walking for 15 minutes five days per week.

Add bike rides with the kids on the weekends.

Find short term goals that are achievable to help you realize what you can accomplish instead of dwelling on what you cannot.

NUTRITION OBSTACLES

Don't:

- Say "I can't stay with the nutritional plan."

Do write down specific issues, like:

- "I always eat too much after dinner."
- "Ice cream gets me every night."

Now you can come up with one or more specific workarounds, like these:

- Allow yourself a small bowl of ice cream two nights per week.
- Brush your teeth after dinner so food won't taste as good.
- Watch TV or work in a room without easy access to food.

Whenever you encounter a significant obstacle on your path to health, whether it's changing

your mindset or making lasting changes in your
movement, nutrition, sleep or stress management,

- ⊙ Be specific.
- ⊙ Take ownership.
- ⊙ Force yourself to come up with at
  least one workaround.
- ⊙ Keep your goals small and
  manageable.

Supplements

In an ideal world, all our nutrients would come from real foods, not pills, as we followed the nutritional plan outlined in this book:

- ⊙ Plant-based, emphasizing a variety of organic vegetables
- ⊙ Whole food, Mediterranean-style
- ⊙ Plenty of monounsaturated fats like avocados, nuts and olive oil,
- ⊙ Appropriate portions of wild or pasture-raised animal products like fish, chicken, meat and cheese.

However, I understand that it can be challenging to eat this way every day. Given our altered soil composition and our industrial feeding practices, even a well-balanced diet can leave you deficient in certain nutrients.

Therefore, I recommend three supplements below that will benefit most people. However, you'll benefit most from individualized supplement recommendations based on factors like your own nutritional habits, where you live, how much time you spend outdoors, your medications, and other factors. If possible, seek out an experienced provider to personalize your supplement plan. And remember, please discuss starting and stopping any medication or supplement with your physician.

OMEGA-3 FATTY ACIDS

Omega-3 fatty acids (O3FAs) have been shown to have numerous health benefits, primarily from specific components called DHA, EPA and ALA. They reduce the risk of death following a heart attack and reduce cardiac arrhythmias. They've also been shown to reduce inflammation, to inhibit platelet inhibition, lower triglycerides, improve endothelial blood vessel health, and stabilize plaque.

DHA and EPA are longer-chain fatty acids found exclusively in seafood and marine algae. ALA, or alpha-linolenic acid, is a shorter chain fatty acid that is found in plant foods such as flax, hemp, pumpkin seeds, and walnuts.

Current research suggests that DHA and EPA are the primary source of health benefits in O3FAs. ALA is also beneficial, although to a lesser degree.

Multiple studies suggest that most modern societies suffer from a lack of omega 3, and an overabundance of omega 6 fatty acids.

Omega-6 fatty acids are also required for multiple functions including building cell membranes and helping repair cells. However, higher levels of omega 6 FAs have been implicated in potentially dangerous functions like promoting inflammation and oxidation.

So even though both omega-6 and omega-3 fatty acids are important for our health, we need to balance the more beneficial omega-3 sources with the potentially harmful (at higher doses) omega-6 sources.

Research has shown that hunter-gatherer societies typically consumed a diet with an omega-6 to omega-3 ratio of 1:1 to a maximum of 3:1. The assumption is that this low ratio of omega-6 to omega-3 fatty acids may explain why these societies have fewer inflammatory diseases.

Modern industrialized Western societies, however, tend to have a ratio of 20:1! This is predominantly from excessive use of safflower oil, sunflower oil, corn oil and soybean oil, all of which are high in omega-6.

In addition, changes in farming and feed techniques have altered our sources of omega-3 fatty acids. Farmed fish contain significantly less omega-3 than wild fish. Soy- and grain-fed livestock and poultry contain much less omega-3 than grass- and pasture-raised animals.

Observational evidence suggests that replacement of anti-inflammatory omega-3s with pro-inflammatory omega-6s may be related to growth in chronic inflammatory diseases such as heart disease, diabetes, cancer and auto-immune diseases.

For instance, why do traditional Japanese men and women have lower rates of inflammatory diseases despite higher rates of smoking and high blood pressure? Studies have shown that their typical diet's omega-6 to omega-3 ratio is more in line with hunter-gatherer societies. Again, it is not causative proof, but it's worthy of further investigation.

The key to correcting the ratio starts with eating less vegetable oil, fewer refined cereal grains like wheat and corn, and fewer processed foods.

It also requires eating more omega-3 dense foods like wild fish, grass-fed meat and eggs from pasture-raised chickens.

Eating in this manner will improve your omega 6-to omega-3 ratio. You'll also improve your overall nutrition.

Regardless of your ratios, this is the smartest way to eat!

Even when we make these nutritional changes, we may still fall short in our omega-3 to omega-6 ratio due to the reduced quality of our animal fats.

That's why I recommend a high-quality omega-3 DHA/EPA supplement for most people.

By "high quality" I specifically mean a supplement that:

- ⊙ Contains at least 500 mg of DHA/EPA combined
- ⊙ Uses a well-absorbed formulation. Triglyceride oil and ethyl ester oil tend to be better than synthetic triglyceride oil
- ⊙ Is manufactured with a detailed distillation process to remove heavy metals and other toxins. ConsumerLab.com is an excellent independent source for advice on product safety and purity.

Quality is of the utmost importance when it comes to omega-3 fatty acid supplements. One of my favorites is Thorne's "Super EPA" supplement. Thorne uses a quality distillation process, their formulation is well-absorbed, and their brand's purity and quality has been well-respected for years. While this brand is slightly more expensive, it's worth a few extra dollars per bottle. I've also had good experience with Vital Choice Wild Salmon Oil. That said, they certainly are not the only high-quality brands out there. Just do your homework before you buy.

Krill oil is another popular form of omega-3 supplementation. Krill are tiny marine creatures. They reside low on the food chain, eating phytoplankton and algae instead of other fish. This means they have less contamination from heavy metals and other toxins. Sardine- and anchovy-based fish oils have naturally lower levels of toxicity for the same reason.

Krill oil also contains a natural antioxidant called astaxanthin, and can be more easily absorbed into the body. However, krill oil is generally more expensive than regular fish oil and comes in smaller doses, so let your budget be your guide.

If you have a shellfish or seafood allergy, discuss which omega-3 supplement is best for you with your doctor.

VITAMIN D

Vitamin D is crucial for bone growth and strength. It works by improving calcium and phosphorus absorption, and studies have suggested, although not definitively proven, multiple other health benefits as well. These benefits include reducing the risk of multiple sclerosis, diabetes, depression, heart disease, and even improving weight loss.

However, despite their multiple potential benefits, it is estimated that over 50% of Americans are deficient in vitamin D. This can, in part, be explained by the difficulty in getting adequate vitamin D from our food. Naturally-occurring Vitamin D is found almost exclusively in seafood, and it takes eight ounces a day of wild fatty fish to provide 2,000 IU of Vitamin D. I'm a big fan of fish, and even I can admit that's a *lot* of fish!

Milk and yogurt are frequently fortified with vitamin D, but not at sufficiently high enough doses to meet our body requirements.

The most efficient way to get vitamin D is not from food at all, but from sunlight. When UVB rays hit our bodies, they convert a cholesterol substance in our skin to vitamin D3. The liver then converts D3 to its active form, 25-hydroxy-vitamin D. This is the substance that most lab tests analyze to measure your vitamin D level.

Thirty minutes of body exposure in the middle of a summer day can provide a pale-skinned person with over 10,000 IU of Vitamin D.

This efficiency is decreased in people with darker skin, with use of sunscreen, in different latitudes, with high levels of pollution and at other times of day or seasons of the year. And of course, prolonged unprotected sun exposure increases the risk of skin cancer.

Therefore, it can be very difficult to get adequate levels of vitamin D even from sun exposure. Traditional hunter-gatherer tribes spend most of their day outside in the sun with minimal barriers on their skin. You can bet they have adequate vitamin D levels. That is clearly not the case in most modern industrialized societies.

Fortunately, it's easy to measure your Vitamin D level and gauge the amount of supplementation needed. Normal ranges can vary, and there is some debate about "optimal" levels. I recommend a goal between 40-60 ng/ml. This seems to be the best balance between optimal levels yet safely avoiding toxicity from too much Vitamin D.

In general, 2000-5,000 IU is an appropriate starting dose. Adjust your supplementation according to your blood test results. Make sure you choose vitamin *D3* supplements, as they are much more efficiently absorbed than vitamin D2.

VITAMIN K2

Vitamin K2 helps keep calcium in the bones and teeth where it belongs, and helps prevent it from going to the blood vessels and soft tissues where it does not belong.

Vitamin K2 is likely the most under-appreciated vitamin that I recommend, but its potential health benefits are starting to get more attention.

Don't confuse Vitamin K2 and Vitamin K1. Vitamin K1 is the most commonly discussed version of vitamin K. It's involved in blood clotting and is found in green leafy vegetables. The commonly prescribed blood thinner warfarin works by inhibiting vitamin K1 and is therefore counteracted by green leafy vegetables.

Vitamin K2, however, is a distinct substance that is important for calcium regulation.

Vitamin K2's history is fascinating. A dentist, Dr. Weston Price, discovered a nutrient that he called "activator x" which greatly improved dental health. This nutrient was later identified as Vitamin K2.

Dr. Price found this nutrient in butter and milk from cows grazing on "rapidly growing" grass and alfalfa, and not from cows grazing on less healthy grass sources.

Not surprisingly, then, the best food sources for Vitamin K2 are grass-fed livestock and egg yolks from pasture-raised chickens. Grain-fed cows and pen-raised hens are inferior at producing foods containing Vitamin K2.

Low-fat diets tend to be severely deficient in vitamin K2, and even high-fat diets can be deficient if the quality of the fats is less than optimal.

For that reason, K2 supplements are very important, specifically the MK-4 version. Clinical trials have shown that the MK-4 version reduces the risk of fractures, which is the best metric for bone health (there is also a MK-7 version but this has not been studied to the same degree as MK-4).

Importantly, Vitamin K2 and Vitamin D3 work synergistically to promote bone health, and potentially to reduce cardiovascular risk. They are a powerful combined supplement.

A good friend of mine, Dr. John Neustadt, has given many excellent talks on this subject. Search for his talks in Google if you want to delve more deeply into Vitamin K2.

There is some controversy as to the exact recommended dose of vitamin K2. I suggest a minimum of 1 mg/day up to 45mg/day.

Warning: Theoretically, Vitamin K2 could potentially interact with Vitamin-K antagonist blood thinners such as warfarin. I have no clinical experience using it with warfarin as I have purposely avoided it. You should consult with your physician prior to starting Vitamin K2 if you are on warfarin or other blood thinners.

Recommended Reading

THE SIX BUILDING BLOCKS OF GOOD HEALTH

Mindset: The New Psychology of Success. Carol Dweck, Ph.D.

This is the "bible" for the concept of mindset. She uses her extensive clinical experience along with scientific research to explain the difference between a fixed mindset and a growth mindset. Full of analogies and explanations of how the growth mindset prepares us for success in multiple areas of life.

Good Calories, Bad Calories: Fats, Carbs, and the Controversial Science of Diet and Health. Gary Taubes.

This is a detailed description from Mr. Taubes, a prolific health writer, about the history of our nutritional patterns. His extensive research shows how much of our nutritional knowledge is misguided and based on poor science.

The Paleo Cure: Eat Right for Your Genes, Body Type, and Personal Health Needs. Chris Kresser.

This is an excellent introduction to the paleo nutritional concept, and the paleo lifestyle as a whole. This book provides a framework for lifestyle as medicine, and is very detailed about the importance of a "paleo-style" nutritional pattern. It is well rooted in science as well as Mr. Kresser's clinical experience. He is not 100% dogmatic about a paleo diet, and emphasizes the concepts over the exact letter-of-the-law.

Pure White and Deadly: How Sugar is Killing Us and What We Can Do to Stop It. John Yudkin and Robert H. Lustig, M.D.

Dr. Lustig revitalizes and updates Dr. Yudkin's 1970s-era work about the dangers of sugar. Eye-opening regarding the prevalence and health dangers of added sugar.

The Big Fat Surprise: Why Butter, Meat and Cheese Belong in a Healthy Diet. Nina Teicholz.

One of the most important books revolutionizing our perceptions of the health risks and benefits of carbohydrates and fats. Ms. Teicholz does an excellent job of uncovering the faults in the reasoning behind the low-fat movement and explains how it has actually harmed us, rather than helped us.

Eat Fat to Get Thin: Why the Fat We Eat is Key to Sustained Weight Loss and Vibrant Health. Mark Hyman, M.D.

Dr. Hyman is one of the most prominent practitioners of functional medicine. In his book, he explains the pitfalls of the low-fat diet and goes into detail about the importance of eating fat not just for weight loss, but for your health as a whole.

The Obesity Code: Unlocking the Secrets to Weight Loss. Jason Fung, M.D.

Dr. Fung is one of the preeminent practitioners of intermittent fasting, and one of the biggest proponents that insulin, not glucose should be the target of our lifestyle and therapies. In this book, he explains how obesity is largely the result of our hormones, specifically insulin, and what we can do about it.

Always Hungry? Conquer Cravings, Retrain Your Fat Cells and Lose Weight Permanently. David Ludwig, M.D.

This book does an excellent job of explaining in detail how our bodies react to the food we eat. It is full of helpful recipes, and it also addresses overall lifestyle changes beyond just food.

The Book of Awesome. Neil Pasricha.

Neil has a way of finding the "awesome" in routine, everyday occurrences. His simplicity and detailed descriptions, appreciating the little things in life, are lessons for us all.

COOKBOOKS

Recommending cookbooks is a tricky endeavor. For one thing, food tastes differ greatly between individuals, and a wonderful cookbook for one person may not be palatable for someone else.

Second, there are plenty of cookbooks that I enjoy and authors I respect, where I can still find a few recipes that I completely disagree with.

And third, there are thousands of cookbooks available that I have never read. I can only comment on those that I know a little about.

With that in mind, here's my short list of favorites.

As you look through them, keep in mind these important concepts

- ⊙ Real foods
- ⊙ Vegetable-based
- ⊙ Healthy fats
- ⊙ High-quality animal proteins
- ⊙ Low sugar
- ⊙ Low refined grains
- ⊙ Minimal processing

Not all the recipes will fit these criteria. But those that do will be worth it! And remember, you can always add high-quality animal proteins to the recipes in vegetarian cookbooks, if you wish.

True Food: Seasonal, Sustainable, Simple, Pure. Andrew Weil, M.D. and Sam Fox.

Fast Food, Good Food. Andrew Weil, M.D.

The Anti-Inflammation Cookbook. Amanda Haas.

The Gluten-Free Vegan. Susan O'Brien.

The Complete Vegetarian Cookbook. America's Test Kitchen.

The Blood Sugar Solution Cookbook. Mark Hyman, M.D.

49259447R00139

Made in the USA
San Bernardino, CA
18 May 2017